The Book of
SUFI HEALING

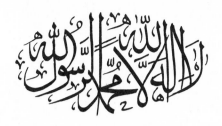

لا إله إلا الله محمد رسول الله

The Book of
SUFI HEALING

Shaykh
Hakim Moinuddin Chishti

Inner Traditions International
Rochester, Vermont

Inner Traditions International
One Park Street
Rochester, Vermont 05767

LIBRARY OF CONGRESS CATALOGING-IN-PUBLICATION DATA

Moinuddin, abu-Abdullah Ghulam.
The book of Sufi healing / Moinuddin Chishti.
p. cm.
Reprint. Originally published: New York : Inner Traditions International, c1985.
Includes bibliographical references and index.
ISBN 0-89281-324-5
1. Sufism. 2. Spiritual healing. 3. Medicine, Arabic. 4. Metaphysics. I. Title.
BP189.65.F35M65 1991
613—dc20 91–14595
CIP

Printed and bound in the United States

10 9 8 7 6 5 4

Text design by Studio 31

Distributed to the book trade in Canada by Publishers Group West (PGW), Toronto, Ontario

Distributed to the book trade in the United Kingdom by Deep Books, London

Distributed to the book trade in Australia by Millennium Books, Newtown, N.S.W.

Distributed to the book trade in New Zealand by Tandem Press, Auckland

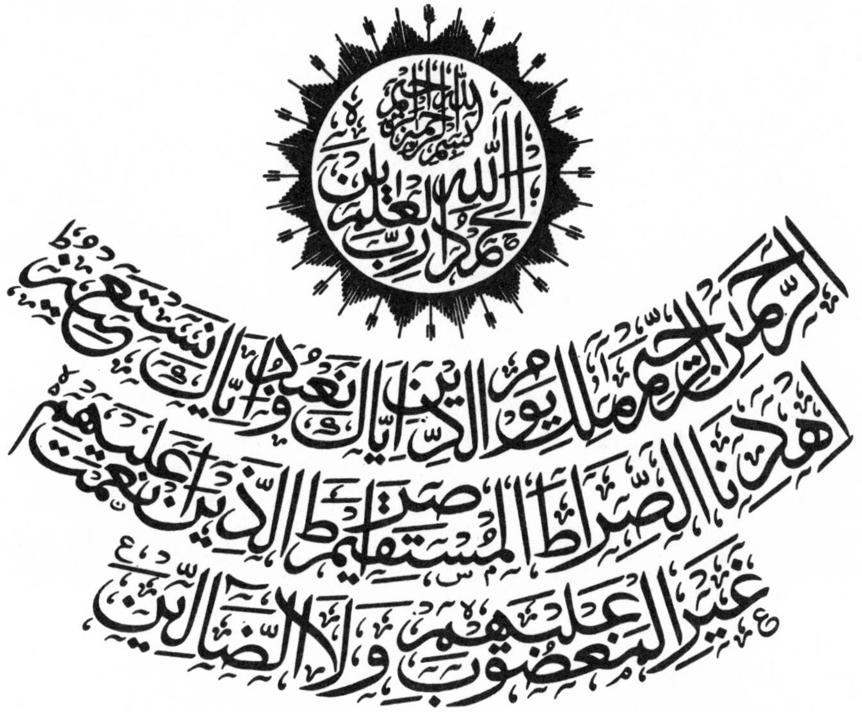

In the name of God, Most Gracious, Most Merciful.

Praise be to God, the Cherisher and Sustainer of the Worlds; Most Gracious, Most Merciful; Master of the Day of Judgment. Thee do we worship and Thine aid we seek. Show us the straight way, the way of those on whom thou hast bestowed Thy Grace, those who have not earned Thine anger and who go not astray.

Contents

Foreword by Abu Anees Muhammad Barkat Ali vii
Shajarah, or Line of Succession, of Shaykh Moinuddin ix
Notes on the Transliteration and Pronunciation of Arabic Words xiii

Preface 1
Prologue 9
1 What Is Health? 11
2 The Hierarchy of Creation 17
3 The Stations of the Soul 25
4 Food and Health 39
5 Akhlāṭ: The Four Essences of the Body 45
6 Foods of the Prophet (s.a.w.s.) 51
7 Herbal Formulas for Common Ailments 65
8 Fasting: The Best Medicine 85
9 Ṣalāt: The Postures of the Prophets 91
10 The Soul of the Rose 111
11 The Universe of the Breath 123
12 Taᶜwīdh: The Mericiful Prescriptions 131
13 Dhikr: Divine Remembrance 141
14 The Origin of Miracles 149
15 The Keys of the Treasures of the Heavens and the Earth 155
16 The Infallible Remedy 159

Appendixes
I. The Islamic Calendar 165
II. Some Useful Short Sūrahs of the Holy Qur'an 167
III. The Divine Attributes 171
IV. Glossary 179
V. Bibliography 183
Index 187

اَلْعِلْمُ عِلْمَانِ عِلْمُ الْأَبْدَانِ ثُمَّ عِلْمُ الْأَدْيَانِ

There are two kinds of Knowledge:
the knowledge of religions and the
knowledge of the body.

مَا خَلَقَ اللهُ دَاءً اِلَّا وَ خَلَقَ لَهُ الدَّوَاءَ اِلَّا الْهَرَمَ

God has not created any illness without
creating also its cure, except old age.

Foreword

Bismillāh, ir-Raḥmān ir-Raḥīm

Not even the highest degree of dedication to worship may earn anybody the claim of divine forgiveness or recompense in any other form, yet there is one thing that everybody should make sure of, which shall not go unrequited under any circumstance by Allah the Almighty, and that is the selfless service to the ailing humanity. There is no other human act more favorably acceptable to Allah than helping the sick and the suffering creatures of His. That is what Shaykh Hakim Abu Abdullah Moinuddin Chishti has endeavored to do in presenting this *Book of Sufi Healing*.

The subject being a difficult and rare one, there are not very many books in this branch of knowledge. Nevertheless it is most heartening to note that the author has taken great pains in bringing out this commendable work by dint of his unshakable trust in Allah and unswerving will to serve the humanity. He displays ample evidence of his vast knowledge in fields of multifarious kinds—theology, mysticism, Islamic Sufism, medicine, hygiene, astronomy, and modern sciences. One wonders at the depth and insight of his knowledge, essentially the result of intensive as well as extensive study in subjects of diverse nature. He takes up different subjects separately and then correlates and coordinates them to converge on a central point, namely health, be it physical and mental health or purification of the soul. This he has done most logically and methodically. What part do *ṣalāt*, fasting, *taᶜwīdh*, or recitation of the Holy Qur'an or *dhikr* of Allah the Almighty in any other form play in physical and mental health or purification of one's *nafs*? The answer is not very far to seek.

The author has also endeavored to dispel doubts and misgivings about Islamic Sufism, a most misunderstood subject in the West. It is a tremendous effort on the part of the author to vindicate the cause of Islam and Sufism. The presentation of additional information in the shape of illustrations, list of herbs with their characteristics and ailments with their treatment, glossary of mystical terms, Qur'anic verses aptly quoted, basic information about *ṣalāt*, fasting, *dhikr*, and so on, has made the book still more beneficial for the ordinary reader. Indeed, *The Book of Sufi Healing* is a blessing for the English-reading world population in general and fellow American and Muslim brethren of the author in particular. In creating such a fine book, the author has rendered a great service to the cause of Islam in the sense that, as Islam is the most natural faith, adherence to its tenets and principles is the only course leading toward human perfection and establishing the rule of Allah the Almighty on this earth. For Sufism in its purest form is nothing else but Islam and Islam only.

I wish the author still more courage and determination to serve the cause of Islam and betterment of the ailing humanity.

Abu Anees Muhammad Barkat Ali

Dar-ul-Ehsan,
Faisalabad,
Pakistan

Shajarah Sharif

of Shaykh Hakim Abu Abdullah Moinuddin

بِسْمِ اللّٰهِ الرَّحْمٰنِ الرَّحِيْمِ

حق —————— حق —————— حق

Allah, The Exalted, The Almighty

Huzur Sar-dār-i-Ka'ināt Muḥammad Muṣṭafā
The Holy Prophet of Islam (s.a.w.s.)

❖

Amīr al-Mu'minīn
Hazrat ᶜAli (r.a.a.)

❖

Hazrat Khwāja Hasan Baṣrī

❖

Khwāja ᶜAbdul-Wāḥid

❖

Fuḍayl ibn Ayaḍ

❖

Ibrahim ibn Adham

❖

Ṣadīq Mar ᶜashī

❖

Ulū Namshād

❖

Abū Isḥāq Shami

❖

Abū Aḥmad Abdāl Chishtī

❖

Muḥammad Zāhid Maqbūl Chishtī

❖

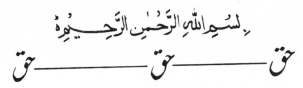

Abū Yusūf Chishtī

❖

Naṣiruddīn Chishtī

❖

Mawdūd Chishtī

❖

Sharif Zindāni

❖

Khwāja ^{c}Uthmān Harūnī

❖

Khwāja Mu^{c}īnuddīn Chishtī of Ajmer

❖

Khwāja Quṭbuddīn Bakhtiyār Kākī

❖

Shaykh Farīduddīn Mas^{c}ūd Ganj-i Shakar

❖

Hazrat ^{c}Alāuddin ^{c}Ali Aḥmad Sābir of Kalyar

❖

Hazrat Shamsuddīn Turk of Panipat

❖

Hazrat Jalāluddīn Mahmūd of Panipat

❖

Hazrat Aḥmad ^{c}Abdul-Haqq Randauli Inkeja

❖

Hazrat Shaykh ^{c}Ārif of Randauli

❖

Hazrat Shaykh Muhammad

❖

^{c}Abdul-Quddūs of Gangoh

❖

Kabir-ul-Awlia Jalāluddīn Farūqī Thanesar

❖

Niẓāmuddīn Balkh Rahnumah

❖

Abū Sa^{c}id Gangohī

❖

Muḥammad Ṣadīq

❖

Muḥammad Da^{c}ūd

❖

Shāh Abūl-Ma^{c}ālī

❖

Muḥammad Sa^{c}id

❖

Sa^{c}id Shah Muḥammad Salīm

❖

Shah ^{c}Inayatullāh

❖

^{c}Abdul-Karīm

❖

Ḥafiẓ ^{c}Abdul-Raḥīm

❖

Hazrat Shāh Hassān

❖

Ḥafiẓ Husayn Shah

❖

Muḥammad Husayn

❖

Muḥammad Murtaza Aḥmad

❖

Sa^{c}id Safdar ^{c}Alī Shāh Chishtī

❖

Hazrat Abu Abdullah Ghulam Moinuddin

❖

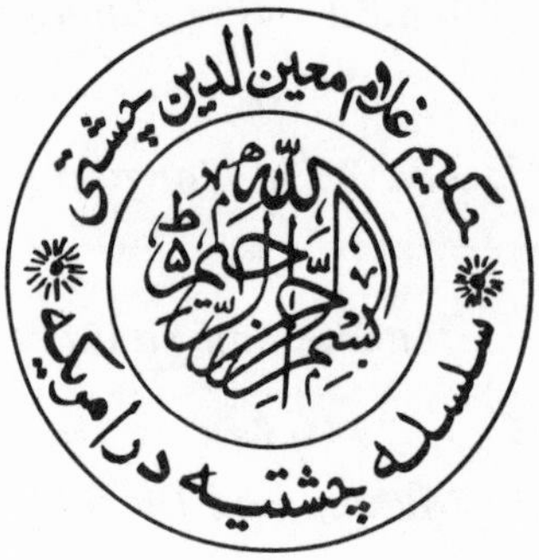

A *shajarah* is the record of the line of succession of a shaykh. It traces the spiritual genealogy from the present shaykh, back in the line to the Prophet Muhammad (s.a.w.s.), who first transmitted the spiritual possessions.

The Sufi genealogy is from the Ṣābiriyyah line of the Chishtiyyah Order of Sufis, headquartered at Ajmer, Rajasthan, India.

Ones who carry on the Sufi teachings are authorized by living shaykhs, who maintain a living link and authority over those below them. This authority is granted by means of formal initiation, and rights of succession are set forth in a Khilāfat-Nama, or Letter of Succession, duly signed and sealed by the senior shaykhs of the order. Hazrat Niẓāmuddīn Awliyā' (r.a.) explained the granting of Khilāfat: "Khilāfat is the right of him who has no aspiration in his mind to have it, and who possesses (1) *ᶜaql salīm* [sound judgment] or matured knowledge to judge all intricate matters of the world with strict impartiality and forbearance; (2) who is an accomplished scholar; and (3) whose chest is full of divine love and wisdom."

The shaykh serves as an indirect link with the Divine Power. The *tabarrukāt muṣṭafawī*—the sacred robes and relics coming down from the line of Chishti shaykhs—are conveyed to the shaykh upon Khilāfat.

Hazrat Abu Abdullah Moinuddin is the twenty-sixth successor in the line of Hazrat Khwāja Muᶜīnuddīn Chishtī (r.a.)

Notes on the Transliteration and Pronunciation of Arabic Words

Arabic consonants are pronounced like English consonants, with the following exceptions.

' A simple stop in the breath.

th Pronounced like *th* in *thin*.

kh Pronounced like *ch* in Scottish *loch* or Yiddish *challah*.

ḥ An *h* sounded with a strong outbreath.

dh Pronounced like *th* in *the*.

r A slightly rolled *r*.

ṣ An emphatic *s* sounded with the tongue at the roof of the mouth.

ḍ An emphatic *d* sounded with the tongue at the roof of the mouth.

ṭ An emphatic *t* sounded with the tongue at the roof of the mouth.

ẓ An emphatic sound between *z* and *dh*.

ᶜ A consonant formed by constricting the back of the throat and pushing the breath outward.

gh A sound like clearing the throat, or like a French *r*.

q A *k* sound from the back of the throat, like the *c* in *court* as opposed to *cat*.

Arabic vowels are divided into long and short. The short vowels *a, i, u* are pronounced as in *cat, fit,* and *duty*. They are not indicated in transliteration by any special marks. The long vowels are about twice as long *in duration* as the short vowels, and are marked as follows:

ā *ah* as in *father*

ī *ee* as in *seen*

ū *oo* as in *you*.

Arabic has two complex vowels: *ay*, often pronounced like *eye* but sometimes as in *bay*, and *aw*, pronounced between *cow* and *boat*.

All prayers and sacred phrases have been transliterated according to a special format that may help the reader with pronunciation. The Names of God are capitalized so as to be easily recognized. *Allāh* begins with a letter whose sound often vanishes with elisions. In such cases the Name is indicated by the capitalization of its first sounded letter: *Llāh*.

Names of ancient shaykhs have been written according to Arabic transliteration. Contemporary shaykhs' spellings have not been standardized. Certain phrases that find their derivation or major usage in Persian, Turkish, or Urdu have not been set in Arabic transliteration style. The same is true of terms that have become common in English.

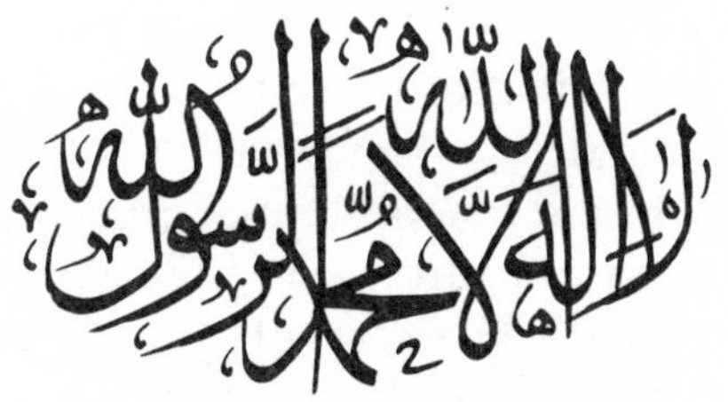

Preface

Bismi Llāh ir-Raḥmān, ir-Raḥīm

Subḥān Allāhi wal-ḥamdu li-Llāhi wa lā ilāha illā Llāh wa Allāhu akbar!

All thanks belong to Allah and all praise belong to Allah and there is no deity except Allah and Allah is Greater (than all that we ascribe to Him).

I wish first to give thanks to Allah, Exalted is He, for the very excellence of His creation, and for His mercies which exist and are bestowed in abundance upon His humanity. His benefits are epitomized in the creation, life, and teachings of all of His prophets (may His blessings be upon them all), and perfected in the form of His last Prophet, the master of humanity, chief of both the worlds, Hazrat Muhammad (peace and blessings of Allah be upon him).

To the extent that Allah should permit and inform me, it is my intention to set forth some of the general and specific principles of human health and well-being as they have evolved within the practices of the mystics of Islam, generally called Sufis in the West. While it is understood that for many readers this book may constitute their first contact with some of these ideas, it is sincerely hoped that even persons of long-standing practice of the way of life called Islam, may find herein confirmation of their faith and belief. *Mā shā' Allāh!* (As it pleases Allah the Almighty!)

There are two main purposes to this book: to reveal the health and healing practices unique to the Sufis, and to give some general idea of the stages and progressions involved in adopting the Sufi life.

Many possible approaches could have been taken with the subject of Sufi healing, which is being presented in English for the first time. It must be borne in mind that Sufism is a specialized topic within the study of Islam, and the healing practices of Sufism is an even more refined subject. Obviously the possible matters which could be discussed would run into tens of thousands of volumes, not one!

Moreover, there is a problem in presenting authentic Sufi practices to a public that has perhaps obtained a distorted view of Sufism up to the present time. It is hoped that those whose impression of Sufism is merely some vague perception about "God and goodness" will learn from this book that it is at once a specific and practical set of guidelines for achieving a high state of human evolution. In any event, the contents of this book are offered as one drop in the divine ocean of knowledge.

Let us try to sort out the many conceptions, definitions, and notions of the term "Sufi." One who has true knowledge of the subject has presented it thusly: There is one immediate condition of the soul (*ḥāl*), called *afghan* in Sufi parlance, which refers to the overwhelming joy and love one feels when confronted with or granted a glimpse of the very presence and reality of God Himself.* One is compelled to shed sweet tears. While this condition no doubt comes and goes, the accounts are not few of pious personalities who were afflicted with this supreme joy for years on end.

A second meaning of the word *afghan* refers to the spiritual station (*maqām*) of the soul, characterized by the one who has achieved true purity. Such a person can be said to have extinguished the flames or burning (*ātish*) of the various appetites of the ego (*nafs*) to such an extent that they can never be rekindled. Anyone enjoying this status may be referred to as a Sufi. More properly, he or she would be called a *walī* (pl. *awliyā'*), meaning "beloved friend of God."

People, particularly in the West, who casually refer to themselves and others as Sufis do not realize the exalted position of those who have attained such refinement through the grace and blessings of Almighty God. In fact, it would constitute a kind of unparalleled arrogance to presume to describe oneself as at the pinnacle of spiritual perfection. Since true Sufis would of necessity exhibit the height of humility and selflessness, it is difficult to locate one who would admit to such a condition.

The founder of the Chishtiyyah Order of Sufis in India, Hazrat Khwāja Mu^{c}īnuddīn Chishtī (r.a.), has spoken of the true Sufi as one who sees no evil, hears no evil, speaks no evil, and thinks no evil.

Although there are more than 150 orders in Sufism, they are all united in one fact: that all participants, from novice to supreme master, are conformed in inward thought and outward behavior to the religious injunctions of Islam, known as *sharī^{c}at*.

Some mistakenly assert that Sufism is separate from Islam, that it is broad and open-minded, whereas Islam is narrow, static, backward, and old-fashioned. Not only is such a concept ignorant, but it does a tremendous disservice to those who are sincerely seeking the right way of living, of guidance to God. To those who may claim that all paths lead to God, He has replied: If you don't know where you are going, any path will do.

*The pronoun for God in Arabic has neither male nor female gender. I use the conventional literate form, *Him*, only because there is no proper genderless pronoun in English, most certainly intending no offense to femininity.

Literally millions of volumes exist which establish beyond any possibility of doubt that Sufism took seed directly from Islam, was nurtured by Islam, and has reached maturity in Islam. Sufism, far from being separate from Islam, is the very soul of Islam expressed in a conceptual framework.*

The Sufis may be considered a special class of teachers within Islam, whose responsibility is to maintain and transmit the hidden, deeper knowledge (*ᶜilm*) contained in the Holy Qur'an. There are the commonly known and understood teachings of the Holy Book—called *muḥkamāt* (sing. *muḥkam*)—which can be understood easily by anyone. Then there are those divine secrets called *mutashābihāt* (sing. *mutashābih*) which were revealed by the Holy Prophet Muhammad (s.a.w.s.) to Hazrat ᶜAlī (r.a.a.), who in turn conveyed this knowledge to others in an oral transmission which has continued up to the present time through the network of Sufi orders, or *silsila*s.

The life of the Sufi is the life of the spirit, a life adjusted and regulated by the clear guidance for humanity provided by God Himself in the Holy Qur'an. Ultimately, the successful one is granted a personal confrontation with, and absorption in, the overwhelming reality of the Creator, Owner, and Sustainer of existence: Allah.

It is important to note that the word *Allah* does not mean "a" god or a Muslim god. Even Arabic-speaking Christians use the word *Allah* for God. We use the word *Allah*, first, because it has never been used to refer to anything except the One God. Further benefits attached to the Arabic letters and sounds will be elucidated in this book, *in shā'Allah* (God willing).

For the Sufis, the supreme object of life is to serve and obey Allah, thereby earning His pleasure. Just as the Creator indiscriminately bestows sun, rain, and love upon all of His creatures, so too does the Sufi strive to love all of humanity regardless of caste, creed, age, sex, color, religion, or national origin.

The stages of Sufism rest upon the premise that by constant recollection and remembrance of Allah, one will, through the grace of Allah, eventually come to be effaced in the One Remembered.

At the headquarters of the Chishti Order in Ajmer, India, there is one street (more like an alleyway) that runs alongside the *dargah*, or resting place, of Hazrat Khwāja Muᶜīnuddīn Chishtī (r.a.). Along that street are sitting perhaps three dozen men and women at any given time, and from all outward appearances they are the outcasts and most despicable beggars of the world. But one look into their eyes will reveal a countenance of supreme joy and peace, of contentment, of complete reliance and trust upon Allah (*tawwakul Allāh*) to provide all that they may need. Whether they eat or do not eat does not matter to them. They cannot even know if they are clean or dirty. Every person who crosses their path, be he criminal or saint, is given

*It is beyond the scope of the present book to deal fully with this issue. The interested reader is referred to Annemarie Schimmel, *Mystical Dimensions of Islam* (University of North Carolina Press), and Dr. Mir Valiuddin, *Contemplative Disciplines in Sufism* (London, East-West).

the same greeting—an expression of unrestricted love for that person and the deepest prayer that the person may receive the mercies and blessings of Allah. Once this condition sets in, there is no end. *Subḥān Allāh! Subḥān Allāh! Subḥān Allāh!*

It was in this same condition that the well-known Sufi Hazrat Mawlānā Rūmī (r.a.) found himself after completing the greatest sequence of mystical poetry in the world, the *Masnavi*. To show that he was completely resigned to the will of Almighty God, and that he lived solely by the permission and favor of God and not by the blood of the human body, Mawlānā, in the presence of a large gathering of notables, called for a physician (*ḥakīm*). When the healer arrived, Mawlānā ordered that incisions be made through all of his veins and the cuts be allowed to bleed until all flowing ceased. When this act was done and no more blood flowed, Mawlānā rose up and, after performing ablutions, entered his rose garden and commenced the ecstatic twirling of the sacred dance. *Mā shā' Allāh! Al-ḥamdu li-Llāh al-Ḥayyu! Al-Qayyūm!*

Hazrat Bābā Farīd Ganj-i Shakar (r.a.), one of the saints of the Chishtiyyah, has said that the first step or stage of Sufism consists in knowledge of and access to the 18,000 created worlds (*ᶜālamīn;* sing. *ᶜalam*). No doubt, to arrive at the threshold of such a state requires a commitment and level of worship that most humans cannot even imagine.

It is related that Almighty Allah has said: "My servant ceases not to seek nearness to Me through special worship, until I make him My favorite, and thus I become the ears wherewith he hears, the eyes wherewith he sees, the hands wherewith he holds, and the feet wherewith he walks."

This "special worship" is taken up in the form of voluntary prayers during the day, and also extended worship and supplications throughout the night. The masters of the true path are united in their insistence that no progress at all can be made without the middle-night superogatory prayers (*tahajjud*).

By combining this special devotion and obedience to Allah, the Sufis unlock the origin of miracles through which they gain access to the attributes of Allah the Almighty, and reflect these qualities in their own character and actions, to the extent possible in human beings.

Just as the most prominent characteristic or attribute of Allah is His compassion for humanity, so, too, do the Sufis strive to spread and bestow this among the people. Of all service to humanity, that which is considered superior is the healing of the sick and suffering. Certainly the great proportion of Sufi shaykhs have been known for their ability to effect results in the realm of healing various ailments. Of course, it is Allah Who does the actual healing, the shaykh being only the agent for the will of Allah, exalted is He!

The Chishtiyyah Order of Sufis, one of the four largest in Islam, has carried on this tradition of serving the downtrodden of humanity—the sick and ailing—for the past eight hundred years, ever since the founding of the order. A large herbal-medicine clinic is attached to the *dargah* premises at Ajmer, and all persons coming there (upward of sixty thousand per day) are provided whatever treatment they need, free of charge or obligation. *Mā shā' Allāh!*

If Allah touch thee with affliction,
none can remove it but He. (Qur'an 6:17)

The above verse forms the basis of this book, which has been written to provide specific means to attain a true health of the body, mind, and soul. For these suggestions to be put into practice successfully requires only the state of being known as *tawwakul Allāh* (trust in Almighty Allah). To inspire the reader's confidence in the suggestions which follow, I have cited examples of various Sufi personages past and present. All of these persons have derived their own example and inspiration from that of the Holy Prophet Muhammad (s.a.w.s.), whose life has been aptly described as "the Qur'an lived."

The physical healing methods of the Sufis derive first from the Qur'an and second from the traditions and actions of the Prophet Muhammad (s.a.w.s.). Furthermore, there are many men and women of brilliance who have developed the knowledges of physical medicine in the context of Islamic societies and culture. Hakīm Ibn Sina, Rhazes, and al-Suyuti are among these medical authorities frequently studied by the Sufis.

I have made little effort to rationalize or otherwise justify the healing claims contained in this book, except to identify their source and origin, which in the end is God. In fact, materialistic ideologies and scientific theories can never be sufficient to explain the divine mysteries. Nonetheless, these practices have proved effective and useful for an untold but very great number of persons and are in current use among the mystics of Islam.

At the same time, it must be noted that what is required for one to attain to the state of being of a *walī* or Sufi—and utilizing the healing methods herein—is not the same thing as reading this book. One who is sincerely interested in taking up a formal curriculum of study in Sufi healing must find an authentic shaykh or master and wholeheartedly submit to the advice offered. Some say that at least twelve years are required for this training.

The health practices fall into three categories: (1) those for the body, (2) those for the mind or emotions, and (3) those for the soul. The best and preferred practices are those for the soul. However, a person whose mind and soul are degenerated or weak, may be unable to act upon or be acted upon by a purely spiritual practice. In such a case, herbal remedies, food restrictions such as dieting and fasting, and similar modes are employed. Practices for the heart are also employed favorably in such cases, for they awaken, enliven, and disseminate various divine potentialities throughout the person.

The practices for the soul are highly charged with divine grace and blessings, and if rightly applied, will never fail to bring results. It is a principle of nature that the spiritual always takes precedence over the material.

My own study of the sciences of Islamic mysticism (*taṣawwuf*) began in 1968 with a written correspondence with my shaykh, the late Hazrat Maulana Sufi Wahiduddin Begg (may Allah grant him the choicest blessings, as many of such things as there are, *āmīn!*). Prior to his demise in Ajmer in February 1979, our exchange of letters had grown to some four thousand pages, which form the corpus of his teachings to me.

During this period it was my good fortune to travel to Afghanistan, where I took up a formal course of study of healing sciences under the guidance of Sufi personages of that beloved land. While there, I was initiated into the healing practices of dream interpretation by Pir Syed Daoud Iqbali, leader of the Naqshbandiyyah Sufis at Dehdadi, near Balkh.

The knowledge of Islamic jurisprudence (*fiqh*) and the science of utilizing various Qur'anic verses in healing (*taᶜwīdh*) were conveyed by Hajji Shaikh-ul-Islam Nimayatullah Shahrani, also while I was in residence in Afghanistan.

In April 1976, while paying my respects to the leader and supreme *murshid* (teacher) of the Chishtiyyah, at the *dargah* of Hazrat Khwāja Muᶜīnuddīn Chishtī (r.a.), I experienced the first of what was to become a continuing sequence of miracles (*karamat*). There, under the direction of my shaykh, I was able to instigate a particular practice that halted a spontaneous abortion which was being suffered by my wife in far-off Kabul—an event that was later termed a miracle even by the attending physicians.

Consequently, I undertook a vow to devote the balance of my life to the duty of serving the humanity, for the sake of Allah Almighty and only for the sake of Allah the Almighty. *Mā shā' Allāh.*

In order to make this volume useful to as many as possible, I have presented wherever I could the original Arabic script as well as the transliteration and translation of various prayers. The words should be uttered in Arabic, for reasons that will become apparent in the following pages.

A special debt of gratitude is hereby acknowledged and expressed for my present shaykh, Syed Safdar Ali Shah Chishti, of Lahore, Pakistan, who has shared with me his spiritual possessions, for which honor and favor I could never adequately express my appreciation.

One of the finest examples and exponents of the ideals expressed in this volume is to be found in the life and personality of Sufi Abu Anees Muhammad Barkat Ali of Dar-ul Ehsan, Pakistan. His miraculous healing experiences are legend throughout the world.

While I was involved in preparing the final typescript of this book, Bernard Glicksberg provided me with great assistance in the mechanical production of the text and allowed me to work unhindered by various external concerns. He proved to be a friend in the truest sense of the word.

The editing of this manuscript was a special challenge. Rabia Harris exerted her knowledge of Arabic in conforming the disparate foreign language elements to one style. And Kendra Crossen discovered many opportunities to clarify and enhance the text. Both of these gracious people earned my respect and gratitude.

The Arabic and Persian calligraphy was contributed by Enayatullah Shahrani, Aishah Holland, Shaykh Shemsuddin Friedlander, and myself. The illustrations were the inspired work of Angela Werneke. A special thanks is due to Leslie Colket, who managed to masterfully coordinate all of the disparate elements of production.

Abu Anees Muhammad Barkat Ali read the manuscript for errors of intent and reason, and Zafar Hussain Khan assisted me by resolving technical matters regarding Sufistic terminology.

My wife, Iman, listened with love and concern to my ideas and efforts while I was writing this book, and I must thank the All-Merciful for her endless support and forbearance.

Finally, I most sincerely thank my publisher, Ehud C. Sperling, president of Inner Traditions International, Ltd., of Rochester, Vermont, for his years of kind forbearance and interest to allow me the time and effort to complete this volume.

May Allah the Merciful reward them all with His choicest blessings! *Āmīn! Āmīn! Āmīn!*

Wa ākhiru da^{c}wānā an al-ḥamdu li-Llāhi rabb il-^{c}ālāmin!
Waṣ-ṣalātu was-salāmu ^{c}alā rasūlihil-karīm!

Rabbanā taqabbal minnā innaka antas-Samī^{c} ul-^{c}Alīm!
Subḥāna Rabbuka rabb ul-^{c}izzati ^{c}ammā yaṣifūn.
Wa salāmun ^{c}alāl-mursalīn.
Wal-ḥamdu li-Llāhi rabb il-^{c}ālamīn!
Āmin!

In the end our claim is that all praise be to Allah, the
Lord of the Worlds, and blessings and greetings to the Prophet (s.a.w.s.).

Our Lord! Accept from us this duty!
Lo! Thou, only Thou, art the Hearer, the Knower!
Gloried be thy Lord, the Lord of Majesty,
From that which they attribute (unto Him)!
Peace be unto His messengers!
Praise be to Allah the Almighty,
Lord of the Worlds! Be it so!

H.M.C.
Dar-ul Iman
Oxford, New York 13830

Prologue

The philosophy of Sufism is best summed up in the words of the final *khutbah* (sermon) of Hazrat Khwāja Muᶜīnuddīn Chishtī (r.a.), which he delivered to his followers just one month before his demise. The great saint said:

Love all and hate none.
Mere talk of peace will avail you naught.
Mere talk of God and religion will not take you far.
Bring out all of the latent powers of your being
and reveal the full magnificence
of your immortal self.
Be surcharged with peace and joy,
And scatter them wherever you are
and wherever you go.
Be a blazing fire of truth,
Be a beauteous blossom of love
And be a soothing balm of peace. With your spiritual light,
dispel the darkness of ignorance;
dissolve the clouds of discord and war
and spread goodwill, peace, and harmony among the people.
Never seek any help, charity, or favors
from anybody except God.
Never go to the courts of kings,
but never refuse to bless and help the needy and the poor,
the widow, and the orphan, if they come to your door.
This is your mission, to serve the people. . . .
Carry it out dutifully and courageously,
so that I, as your Pīr-o-Murshid,
may not be ashamed of any shortcomings on your part
before the Almighty God and our holy predecessors
in the Sufi order [*silsilāh*]
on the Day of Judgment.

In the following pages, my own humble effort is offered to fulfill this pious advice. It is for all people, and constitutes an expression of my unyielding love for the life and example of our beloved leader, the Prophet of Islam and savior of humanity (s.a.w.s.).

If you find the spiritual sparks herein to become uplifted, all praise, thanks, and appreciation belongs to Allah *subḥānu wa taʿalā*, the All-Merciful, the All-Compassionate.

If there be mistakes or errors, the responsibility is entirely my own, and I ask pardon and forgiveness of my Lord.

1

What Is Health?

For you God subjected all that is in
the heavens
And on the earth, all from Him.
Behold! In that are signs for people who
reflect.

Qur'an 45:18

What is health? When we talk about the human organism existing in a state of health, we must first of all understand several interrelated questions.

What is a human being? How did it come into existence? How is it sustained in existence? And what is the purpose of human life? Without understanding the answers to these questions (or at least the questions), we can never have a satisfactory knowledge of the real type of health we should be seeking. For without any criteria for what constitutes the proper functioning of a human being, how can we say that it even matters whether we are ill or well? Just because something feels "good" does not necessarily mean it is of ultimate benefit to us. And conversely, simply because at the moment we seem to have pain, we cannot dismiss this experience as "bad," unless we understand how and what the result of these momentary sensations will be.

Allah says in the Qur'an, "There may be a thing decreed for you that you do not like that is good for you; and things that you like that are not good for you." The great Sufi Imam al-Ghazzalī (r.a.) expressed this idea as follows: "Illness is one of the forms of experience by which humans arrive at a knowledge of God; as He says, 'Illnesses are my servants which I attach to My chosen friends.'"

Thus, we ought not necessarily to consider illness our enemy; rather, we may see it as an event, a mechanism of the body, that is serving to cleanse, purify, and balance us on the physical, emotional, mental, and spiritual planes. Considered from this perspective, a bout of flu, a cold, diarrhea, even some kinds of agonizing pain are friends, enabling our bodies to purge unwanted and potentially harmful toxic by-products of metabolism.

Western medicine endeavors to halt or impede the various eliminative functions of the body—to stop the urge to vomit with stomach remedies; to block diarrhea with potions; to end fever with aspirin and related drugs. Behind every natural action of the human body is an inherent wisdom, a mechanism that allows the body to heal itself. In fact, no herb, food, or any other substance or procedure can do anything on its own to heal; it can only aid and assist the body in its own self-healing role. If your finger is cut, it is not the stitches or the bandage or the iodine that causes it to heal; it is the skin itself that performs this miracle.

When we think of illness, we almost always first think of injury or acute pain as the first stage. But today many people are realizing that other aspects of our mental world, our feelings and thoughts, can become unbalanced and cause illness and suffering, even though there may be nothing clinically "wrong" with a person. This approach to health and disease has come to be known as "holistic."

It is rather easy to understand the physical level. The body lets us know—by means of our sense perceptions—sight, sound, touch, taste, and smell—and the vegetative faculties—when something is wrong, and we take steps to correct the problem. The seat of the vegetative function—that is, the instinctive, life-sustaining work of the body—is the liver, sometimes called the Wheel of Life. All of our physical functions are cued by the functions and enzymes of the liver.

In Arabic, *nafs* is the word for the body and its appetites. *Nafs* means all of the demands of the body—for food, for warmth, for fame and fortune (all of these include emotional needs or drives). All physical diseases can be marked out by one or more of these physical dimensions.

The word *nafs* has many meanings: breath, animal life, soul, self, a person, essence, and more. In Sufism, the progression of the soul is described by considering the evolution of the *nafs*, which manifests in human behavior as one's entire character, personality, and behavior. The *nafsī am-marā* is the commanding soul, which creates inordinate appetites. This is the condition of the *nafs* referred to when one occupies the station of egotism (*maqām an-nafs*).

The behaviors recommended in the Qur'an (*shariᶜat*) are meant to control and subdue these inordinate appetities, leading the *nafs* to a more refined status. The soul that has been entirely purified is called *nafsī kull*, meaning "universal soul," which unites with Allah in the final stage of Sufism. However, even at the latest stages of Sufi practice, one cannot assume oneself to be immune to the blemishes of the soul.

The second aspect of our existence is the mind world, or let us say the emotional and mental world. The mind is not entirely separate from the physical body, but is part of and intimately connected with physical functioning. Moods and feelings that originate in the mind frequently have an effect on the body—emotions such as anger, fear, or extreme joy. When one or more of these is experienced, the blood pressure may rise or fall, the body sweats, tears may come.

Interestingly, some ailments or conditions that we have come to regard as purely emotional have their origin in physical imbalances. An example is severe anger. Psychologists would usually attribute this to a condition of the mind or emotions. But according to the Ṭibb system of the Persian physician Avicenna, severe anger is one of the body's most effective ways of dispelling excess moisture in the area of the heart. It is easily corrected with diet.

The realm of the mental world is called *fikr* in Arabic. In essence, *fikr* means meditation or deep-thought process.

The third component of our existence is the soul, called the *rūḥ*. The *rūḥ* is that which exists after death, which marks the end of both physical and mental life.

The interaction of the three realms (or the activation of the physical and mental realms by the soul realm) is carried out by means of the spirit. Many people use the words "spirit" and "soul" to mean the same thing, yet they are distinctly different and separate. The spirit is what activates the physical-level existence, including thought processes. The word for this spirit-activator is *nafas*. It is activated at the point of the breath. The point of the lips where in-breath and out-breath unite is the link between life and death.

We can live without mental activity and without physical movement. But without breath, life ceases in a very short time. There are people who live without mental existence. Although an electroencephalograph shows that their brain waves are not functioning, they may be kept "alive" by mechanical means. They are called "brain dead," yet they are still regarded as living; we do not bury them. This means that there is something superior to this mental existence and physical existence. Such persons still have something left of life in them, and that something is the breath.

The Sufis consider that the breath of life exists and continues by virtue of the *idhn*, or permission of God, the One Who has created us all. What we call the Creator—God, Allah, Yahweh, or whatever—does not matter. In His ultimately reality, God is one. He gives His permission for human life to exist in the first place, and as long as that permission remains, we may draw breath in and out. Regardless of which system of healing we may wish to apply, or how skilled the practitioner, even if all the healers of the world came together, they could not counteract the *idhn*. When the permission is withdrawn, there is no more breath; life ceases.

Interesting cases bear this out. When a child is born, it does not breathe right away. Some say the shock of the cold air starts it breathing. But not in every case does this happen. The Sufis would say that Allah sends His *idhn* for that particular life to commence. If He does not send His permission, no amount of spanking or technological effort can force the baby to breathe. It will be a stillborn.

On the other hand, sometimes, despite every effort to end a life, the permission overrides human efforts. A recent article in a medical journal told of a couple who had informed their doctor that they did not want to have children under any circumstances. The doctor suggested that the husband undergo a permanent vasectomy, and so it was performed. A few months later the couple was back, furious with the doctor, because the wife had become pregnant. The doctor then offered to perform a free abortion to terminate the pregnancy. This procedure was done. Another month later, the couple sued the doctor for malpractice when the woman discovered that she was still pregnant!

Despite the sterilization and the abortion, the *idhn* of God was that this particular child would be born. And so it was. Clearly, there is an Authority against Whom we have no real ability to interfere.

Consider the nonmanifest realms—the world of dreams, of intuition, of abstract phenomena—and the many cases of people reporting encounters with UFOs, demons, poltergeists, and the like. No one in the West has so far come forward with a fully developed conceptual framework with which to deal with these "other-worldly" experiences. The Sufis use the term *ghayb* to refer to events that transpire in the unseen realms. This unseen realm includes the actions of the soul.

The center, or seat, of the soul's existence is the heart. With what do we associate the heart and soul? Love, compassion, sympathy, mercy, and all of our religious sentiments. When someone dies, the grief of the survivors is felt in the heart. It is actually a physical pain. The heart aches. There is so much terminology in our language about these soul-related aspects of the heart. And no one can deny that these feelings of love and compassion do exist. No one is without them.

In Arabic, the heart is called *qalb*. The heart according to the Sufis is not just a physiological pump for dispersing blood about the body. It serves two more vital, interrelated functions. One, the heart is the storehouse of divine attributes; and two, it is the seat of manufacture of the *nafas*—that life-activating force which enters with each breath, the breath that activates all physiological functions.

Thus, when the *idhn*, or permission of God, is drawn in, it goes immediately to the heart. In some manner, this *idhn* activates all of the divine attributes in various combinations, and these then are carried out into the body.

The Qur'an informs that these divine attributes are approximately ninety-nine in number and are what Allah uses as the means of allowing the human to function and work on the created plane of being.

For example, one of these attributes is called *al-Baṣīr*, which means "the Perceiver." In other words, Allah sees everything at all times; there is nothing that escapes the view of God, not even the most intimate thoughts. This *baṣīr* exists as a potentiality within us at all times, stored in the heart.

When Allah sends His *idhn* in on a breath, and this is combined with certain sounds we utter, the potentiality will then travel through a semigaseous network called a humor. The potentiality moves along this network until it reaches the moist, crystalline lens of the eye. Once there, the potentiality unites with the physical part of the body and becomes the actuality of sight.

Perception, the total potentiality of al-Baṣīr, also includes such things as insight, our sensation of majesty when viewing a panoramic sunset, and similar experiences. All of these perceptive capabilities are included within the potentiality of perception.

All of these ninety-nine divine attributes, then, are stored within the heart. These potentialities may be activated by means of various sounds we utter in combination to make words.

The three basic sounds are the long vowel sounds of *ā, ī,* and *ū*. These are what the Sufis call the universal harmonic constants, and they are similarly used in all mystic paths that utilize sounds (otherwise called *mantra*s or *waẓīfah*s).

We do not sing or chant these sounds. Rather, they are voiced in the normal course of our conversations. The word *Allāh*, as an example, is just an elongation of the long vowel sound of *ā*, interrupted once with the consonant of the letter *l*, which makes the shape of the letter *ā* with the tongue. Even animals utter various combinations of these three long vowel sounds. The owl, for example, says, "Hoo!" The pronoun for God in Arabic is *Hū*, pronounced exactly the same way that the owl utters its remembrance of the divine name.

Allah has informed us, "Every creature in the Heavens and the earth glorifies His Name." The Sufi, knowing the Arabic tones and names of God, is able to attune to a cosmic conversation that is constantly going on throughout all of existence as countless creatures utter their variations of the divine name.

The use of these three constants is not arbitrary. The long vowel sound of *ā* (as in *father*), as a vibratory tone, travels downward and slightly to the left from the throat and centers in the heart, thereby stimulating all of the divine attributes stored within. The long sound of *ī* (as in *machine*) moves in the opposite direction, up the nasal septum, and vibrates at the point of the pineal gland, which is considered to be a remnant of the third eye, a light-sensitive organ.

The long sound of *ū* (as in *you*) exists when uttered exactly at the point on the pursed lips, the point of connection between the in- and out-breaths. It is where our action meets and intermingles with the divine permission, the *idhn*.

The Sufis use various formulas or combinations of these tones to produce electrifying effects that are able in and of themselves to unlock congested areas within the heart, thereby releasing one or more potentialities. This alone accounts for a considerable number of miraculous cures.

So the very words we use to make conversation are hardly a random matter. When we say the word "eat" (making the sound of the long ī), for example, we are actually stimulating the endocrine system's pineal gland! The pineal gland receives a vibratory signal that causes a series of ethereal shocks which go throughout the body, providing information to all of the physiological functions.

These events are in conjunction with what transpires throughout nature when the sun sends certain germinative shocks through the soil which cause the seed to open and send out rootlets. The germinal center of the seed is activated by shocks from the sun. Likewise, various centers within the human body are awakened by the undulations of the vibratory tones in these universal harmonic constants. The effects upon human health are profound.

This interconnection between the physical and spiritual realms exists all through nature, of which humans are a part. One might say that animals are more attuned to it; sometimes horses and other animals give a particular sound just before they die, and animals nearby know the meaning of this sound. Animals have greater awareness of the unseen realms. Humans should have this knowledge, but they do not seek it. Humans are more bound to the physical plane.

There must be a knowledge and consideration of the physical, mental, and spiritual planes of existence for there to be true health. By understanding each of these planes of being, we can arrive at the correct modes of balancing and treating each one. If the subject of disease is looked into deeply enough, the origin of all illness can be said to lie in the mind. There must be a thought or concept of an illness in order for it to exist. But what is the mind? Some say it is a collection of cells that have many functions and possibilities. But the Sufis attribute a great deal more to the mind, as the repository of the intellect, which God has given to humans, thus making them unique among all of the creation. Before this mind can be adequately understood, we first have to have a conception of the entire universe, from the most minute bacterial life up to God. This is known as the hierarchy of creation.

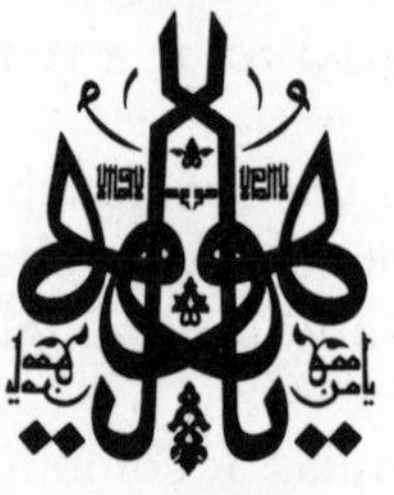

2

The Hierarchy of Creation

God is the One Who created for you
All that is on the earth.
Moreover, He turned to the heaven and fashioned seven heavens with harmony.
He is full of knowledge of all things.

Qur'an 23:17

The hierarchy of creation extends from the most minute forms of terrestrial life up to Allah. The construction of this hierarchy was designed by Allah and is kept in form and balance by His will. In general terms, the whole of creation is divided into two parts: the known world of our human creation (*insān*) and the unseen (*ghayb*) and generally unknown world of the heavens.

The world below, as it were, is the sublunary world, consisting of four elemental spheres: the terrestrial, vegetative, animal, and human kingdoms. These four components are arranged in ascending order of creation, so that the human being occupies the highest position in the order of the physical creation. This dimension is governed by the rules of nature, which is to say the dominion of growth and decay, of life and death.

Above this created world of human existence lies the realm of the heavens, which are eleven in number. Each of these heavens is occupied by angelic forms and ultimately is populated with souls that depart from human bodies and earthly existence.

The various realms of earth and the heavens can be represented in their entirety in the accompanying chart.

Each of the elemental spheres—the terrestrial, vegetable, animal, and human kingdoms—is composed of two parts: an elemental sphere and an interspace, with which it connects to the sphere above its own. Thus, the terrestrial sphere connects with the second elemental sphere via the in-

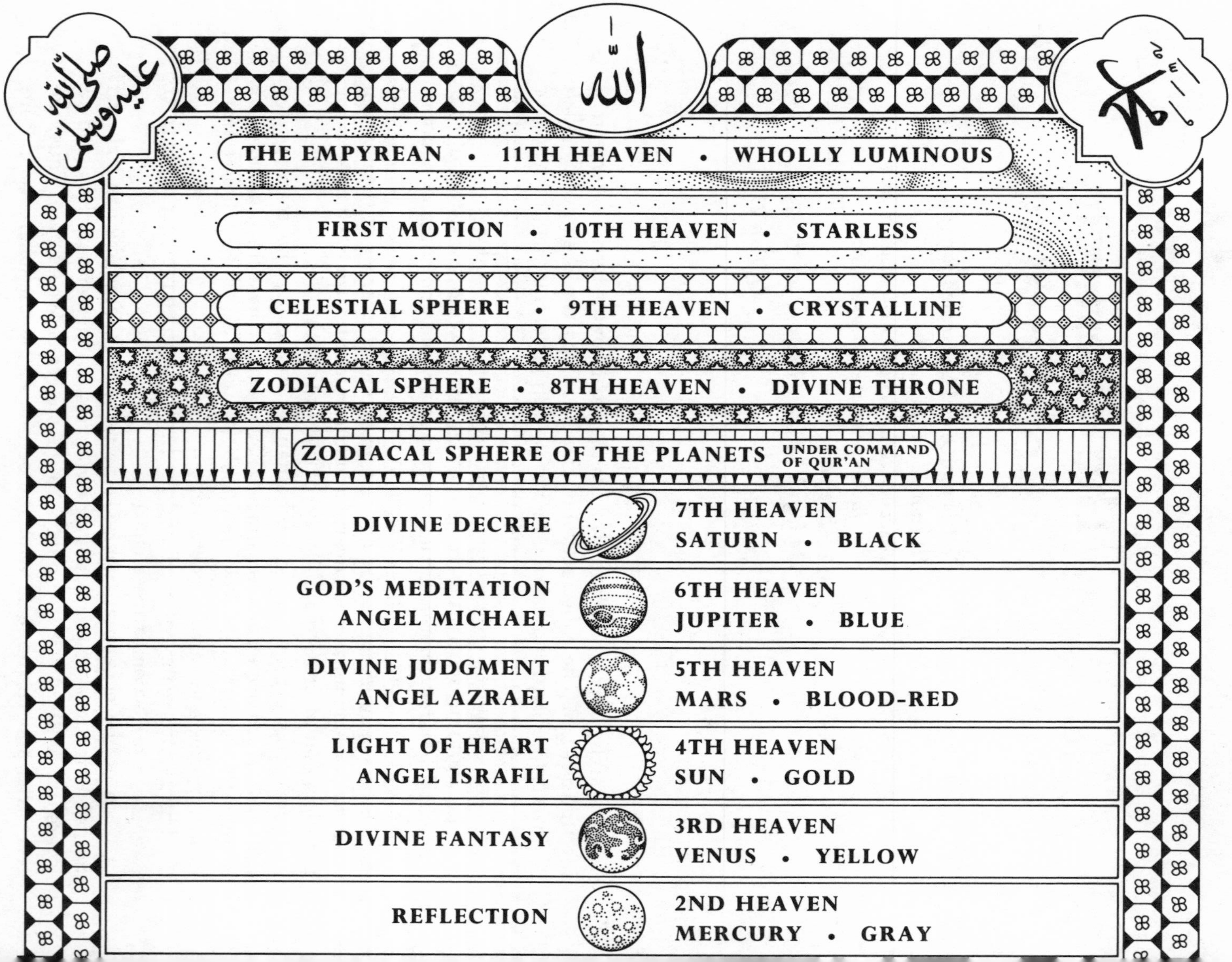
صلى الله عليه وسلم
الله
محمد
THE EMPYREAN • 11TH HEAVEN • WHOLLY LUMINOUS
FIRST MOTION • 10TH HEAVEN • STARLESS
CELESTIAL SPHERE • 9TH HEAVEN • CRYSTALLINE
ZODIACAL SPHERE • 8TH HEAVEN • DIVINE THRONE
ZODIACAL SPHERE OF THE PLANETS UNDER COMMAND OF QUR'AN
DIVINE DECREE
7TH HEAVEN
SATURN • BLACK
GOD'S MEDITATION
ANGEL MICHAEL
6TH HEAVEN
JUPITER • BLUE
DIVINE JUDGMENT
ANGEL AZRAEL
5TH HEAVEN
MARS • BLOOD-RED
LIGHT OF HEART
ANGEL ISRAFIL
4TH HEAVEN
SUN • GOLD
DIVINE FANTASY
3RD HEAVEN
VENUS • YELLOW
REFLECTION
2ND HEAVEN
MERCURY • GRAY

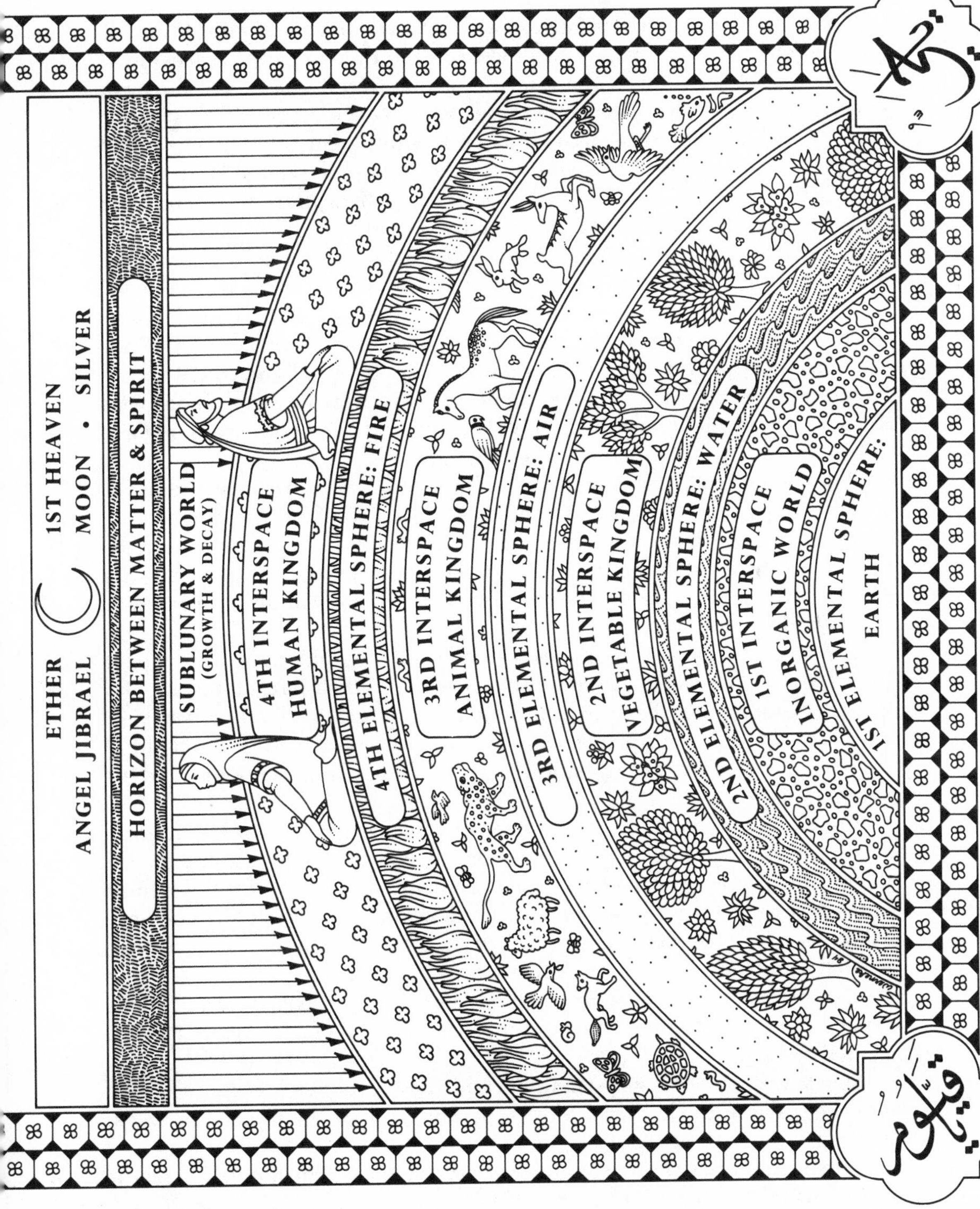
ETHER
1ST HEAVEN
ANGEL JIBRAEL
MOON • SILVER
HORIZON BETWEEN MATTER & SPIRIT
SUBLUNARY WORLD
(GROWTH & DECAY)
4TH INTERSPACE
HUMAN KINGDOM
4TH ELEMENTAL SPHERE: FIRE
3RD INTERSPACE
ANIMAL KINGDOM
3RD ELEMENTAL SPHERE: AIR
2ND INTERSPACE
VEGETABLE KINGDOM
2ND ELEMENTAL SPHERE: WATER
1ST INTERSPACE
INORGANIC WORLD
1ST ELEMENTAL SPHERE:
EARTH

organic world. When the element of water is combined with the terrestrial sphere, the vegetative world is created.

Likewise, the addition of air to earth and water creates fire. When all these combine—earth, water, air, and fire—the human form is made up.

The human kingdom is the interconnection to the heavenly realms. For most humans, the first heaven is represented by the moon: We first attain our strivings for the heavenly realms by viewing the moon. For those who occupy the dimension of the first heaven, or moon, the moon is the firmament and the second heaven represents a higher aspiration—Mercury is their heaven. And so on, up the hierarchy of the heavens.

Humans occupy the highest place in the realms of created life, by virtue of one reason only: Humans have been endowed with the faculty of reason, *ᶜaql*. The *ᶜaql* is the creative, rational reasoning power of the mind, which neither plants nor animals nor water has. These lower forms can only obey their instincts provided by the Creator. They are totally obedient to the laws of nature. For example, one can never "reason" with a deer. If one tries to approach one, it almost invariably bolts instantly and disappears, regardless of the intent of the approaching human.

This holds true even for those animals that humans have sought to control. Dogs, for example, have not taken well to efforts to domesticate them. The more inbreeding that has occurred in a particular breed, the more neurotic the dogs become. Despite efforts to make dogs into pets, it is not so infrequent that a dog will for no reason turn wild upon a person or small child and kill him.

Animals that have been domesticated usually lose the natural dignity of their species. Animals of all kinds are marvelous in their natural terrain. But in that element they have intact all of their natural instinctive behavior, which is required for their survival. The lion does not kill in the wild out of malice. To be a killer is the position given to the lion in the creation, and the lion must do it.

Only humans have the capacity for creative reasoning, for the rational decision-making process by which we decide whether we are going to do a thing. This process is sometimes called free will. One can inform a human being that to do something dangerous will kill him; yet the human being—using his free will—can act contrary to all the evidence and do it anyway. Animals have no such choice: A fish must be a fish.

Our mental decisions are accomplished by the *ᶜaql*, and it is by virtue of this faculty alone that humans have been placed over all of the creation of the sublunary world.

When we aspire to something beyond the earthly existence, we move into the realm of the heavens. Most apparent to all are the zodiacal heavens, which are seven in number.

This is the realm of the planets, the first of which is the moon. Its color is white and silver, and it is constructed from the four elements mentioned, plus ether.

The second zodiacal planet is Mercury, whose color is gray. God said that He made Mercury with the addition of His own *fikr*, His own deep meditative thought.

Venus is the third zodiacal planet, and its color is yellow. Venus governs the world of similitudes, of analogies and metaphors, of poetry. Allah has informed us that Venus was created with the addition of His *khayal*, or imagination.

The sun, the fourth zodiacal planet, is presided over by Israfīl, the Angel of Resurrection. The Prophet (s.a.w.s.) is reported to have related that Israfīl told him that the Angel of Death scans the faces of seventy thousand people each day and, from these, chooses those who will be called from earthly existence. This planet God made from the light of His own heart, the fount of God, the absolute of the heart: love.

The fifth planet in the zodiac is Mars. Its color is blood-red. Azrael, the Angel of Death, presides over this planet, which is created from God's *waḥm*, or divine decision.

Jupiter is the sixth planet of the zodiac, presided over by the archangel Michael and formed of the Light of Himmah—the light of Allah's reflection.

The final zodiacal planet is Saturn. Its color is black. Saturn, being the highest in the hierarchy, was the first zodiacal constellation to be created.

These first seven heavens (presented in reverse order, from lowest to highest) are descriptively named *samā'*. The word *samā'* (heaven) is linked by sound to *samā^c*, an Arabic word meaning "ecstatic contemplation." Each heaven exists with a relation to both something above and something below itself.

These heavens are inhabited by various beings of the creation. There are disembodied souls (having died already to earth life and awaiting the *yawm al-qiyāmmah*, or Day of Judgment) in one or other of the heavens. All the angels exist in all of these various heavens, depending upon their function and rank.

In addition to human souls and angels, Allah also created jinns. Whereas He created humans from the four elements of earth, water, air, and fire, He made the jinns from "smokeless fire." The jinns, which are described fully in the Holy Qur'an, can from time to time assume human form. Generally, they are harmless or favorably inclined to humans, but they can be malevolent. They have great effect upon human affairs and frequently cause imbalances that we would identify as disease. A prime example is colic in infants, who are especially prone to the influence of jinns. Certain herbal substances and recitations are used to dispel jinns.

When the soul is extracted from human life, it begins to ascend through these heavenly realms. So a person would always have consideration of a prior state, and also something to look forward to. This is the reality of the heavenly existence. Those who believe in reincarnation have arrived at their concepts by only partially understanding the entire creation of the heavens.

When we arrive at the highest heaven of the zodiac, we are at the threshold of the Throne of Allah, called the *ᶜarsh*. This is actually a metaphorical statement, as no one could imagine sitting in or anywhere near the seat of Almighty Allah. This eighth heaven constitutes the limit of the physical confines of our universe. The universe we study with telescopes, laser beams, and radio waves reaches its limit at this point of the eighth heaven. Although science has not arrived at this barrier yet, it may in time, God willing.

There are 18,000 created universes, of which we know about only one, the one we inhabit. The other 17,999 exist contiguous to our own and have other functions that we do not know about and never will. Allah has said that He did not create humans with the capacity to totally understand all of His creation. But at the moment of death, when the veils are torn away, each person will instantly see the whole nature of the heavens and the universe and will be astonished at the ingenuity of God's design. Incidentally, Allah has said that despite the complexity of the heavens, He has created the human body infinitely more complex! But for now we shall have to be content to know that there is unimaginable vastness. This inspires us to accept the majesty and power of our Creator, Who has insisted upon many thousands of dimensions of creation; we humans see only one drop in this divine cosmic ocean.

The events of the eighth heaven are directed by Allah Himself; in the lower realms, Allah directs intermediaries to accomplish His designs. When events like shooting stars and meteorites occur in our zodiac, they are caused by actions in this ninth heaven. The regular orbiting of our fixed planets in the earthly heavens is regulated from this heaven.

The ninth heaven is the Crystalline, called the *ᶜarsh*, meaning the Throne of Allah, the dazzlement of God's glory. This state of existence is totally beyond conception or description. A great Sufi once said, "He who climbed over the wall to the *ᶜarsh*, no one ever heard of him again."

The tenth heaven contains no planets or stars and thus is called the Starless Heaven. It is where the motions of all the other spheres originate, directly under the command and decision of Allah the Almighty.

The eleventh heaven is called the Empyrean, or the Heaven of Heavens. It is wholly luminous, nothing but pure, complete, overwhelming light. Mawlānā Rūmī (r.a.) celebrated this realm when he wrote: "What do we care for the Empyrean and the skies? Our journey is to the Rose Garden of Union."

Allah has informed us in the Qur'an that when He decided to make the creation, the first thing He made was the soul of prophecy. And, this, He said, He made from His own light, or *nūr*. In other words, for all of the prophets Allah sent to earth with information for human beings about the nature of the creation, God made for them one soul only. He put this in 120,000 successive human forms, both male and female, some known to the world, some not. Allah made this unimaginably elegant soul from His *nūr*,

His own light. That is why the prophets were able to have such amazing effect upon the world: Allah gave them the powers of illumination over the world.

Allah further said that "If I had not created the soul of prophecy, I would not have created the world." After Allah created this soul of prophecy, it was so brilliant and luminous that it began to perspire. And from this perspiration of the soul of prophecy, Allah made the soul of the rose. This is why the rose has such a magnificent essence and is called the mother of scents. Anyone who looks at a rose smiles and is uplifted, and people all over the world honor and caress the rose instinctively. Indeed, the rose is the symbol of love itself.

We can see from this chart or pathway of the evolution through the hierarchy of creation that humans occupy a relatively low point in it all; there are many levels above that we cannot reach with the physical body. After the earthly, terrestrial life, there are many additional stages, which of necessity must be traversed using the vehicle of the soul. There is a stage beyond the Heaven of Heavens, past the Empyrean, called *wiṣāl*, or the wedding to God Almighty. This alone is the goal of the true Sufi and the real meaning of *Lā ilāha illā Llāh*—that one is content with nothing except the ultimate and final union with the Beloved, the Owner, Creator, and Sustainer of all the Worlds. *Yā ḥayyū! Yā qayyūm!*

Every scripture and every prophet from the first have said the same thing: that we are created by a wise and loving Creator, and that the special purpose of our existence is to endeavor to work our way back to Him. Our objective in life is to regain union with God, and everything in our life is an immense pageant designed to assist us in that journey. That is why one who is active on the Sufi path is referred to as *sālik*, the traveler.

Everything we consider to be kind, good, and desirable in this life is but the minutest manifestation of the final, absolute, and incontrovertible actuality of those things which are owned by Allah and not by anyone else. This final and ultimate knowledge about all things is called *ḥaqīqat* (from *ḥaqq*, truth).

When we speak of love and say we want to be loved or to love someone, what we mean is that we yearn for that absolute love that will overwhelm us and burn us to ashes so that we die of love. One human cannot provide such majestic power of love for another. It is only the Divine Beloved who can annihilate us. That is what the Sufi seeks, or dies trying to achieve.

The journey from a confused, earthly person to one united forever with the Divine Reality is a long, complex, and difficult journey. Therefore, the Sufis have elaborated the various stages on this path and have developed various signposts and measures that can be used to identify where one is on the path. This chart of progression on the journey to the Beloved is called the stations of the soul.

3

The Stations of the Soul

In its progression through life, the physical body passes through stages, from infancy to youth, adulthood, and old age. Similarly, the soul passes through specific evolutionary stages or stations.

The Arabic word for such a station is *maqām* (pl. *maqāmāt*). It means a stopping or resting place. But it has many other connotations that convey the full sense of what this stage may be: place of residence, dwelling, mansion, stay, dignity, office, state, musical tone, question. Indeed, the occupation of a *maqām* by the soul is all of these, and sometimes more.

The stations of the soul are entered into at the moment of birth, and the entire period of life is occupied in one of these stations, although there may be changes from one station to another. These are listed in ascending order as follows:

***Maqām an-Nafs*:** The Station of Egotism

***Maqām-al-Qalb*:** The Station of the Heart

***Maqām-ar-Rūḥ*:** The Station of the Pure Spirit

***Maqām as-Sirr*:** The Station of Divine Secrets

***Maqām al-Qurb*:** The Station of Proximity (or Nearness) to Allah

***Maqām al-Wiṣāl*:** The Station of Union (sometimes called the Divine Wedding with the Beloved)

From the moment of birth, we are constantly striving to develop the soul, and progress in this effort can be marked out and measured by referring to these stages. Obviously, not everyone attains all of the stages. It is important to realize that it is not the body as such that makes this journey, but rather the *rūḥ*.

The translation of *rūḥ* is usually given as "soul." It can also mean the breath of God, the angel Gabriel, the Qur'an, revelation, or prophecy.

For the Sufis, the *rūḥ* is the essence of life. It is not the physical body or the brain and its thoughts and memories; nor is it the life processes. The *rūḥ* has a distinct existence of its own, which is derived from God and belongs entirely to God.

When we ask someone what a pomegranate tastes like, he may well say something like, "It tastes what it tastes like." That does not seem a very satisfactory answer, but because the pomegranate is unique, its taste cannot be related to anything else, hence this curious reply. And so it is with the *rūḥ*.

The *rūḥ*, or essence, can be shown to exist only in relation to rhythm and motif. Think of dance as an example. There is such a thing as dance, but it does not exist concretely except in relation to the form of rhythm and motif. One can imagine a dance with the mind, but for the dance to be actual, the motion and rhythm of dancers are needed to act it out. But the dance remains the essence. This is what is meant by essence, of which the *rūḥ* is perhaps the supreme example.

The human soul also requires this rhythm and motif to be manifest on the physical plane. Remember that the *rūḥ*, or soul's essence, is not the same thing as the spirit (*nafas*). The latter is the divine force that activates the physical phenomena in the body, including mental processes. The *rūḥ* is more intimately felt and superior to the spirit.

Imagine all of the things that have the essence of fire in them—the sun, green wood, ashes, and so forth. All have the same essence, but they possess very different physical forms, and each is at a different stage of evolution, a different *maqām*. The absolute of the essence of fire is part of the *nūr*, or light of God.

Every physical created thing has its unique and characteristic balance—between hot and cold, moist and dry, passivity and activity. We read in the Qur'an that Allah "has created everything in its correct balance." For example, the blood is characteristically warm and moist. Anything that disturbs or changes that normal balanced condition may lead to disease. The same is true of our emotions. Our moods are constantly affected by events coming in via our sensory apparatus. Take the sense of touch. If someone slapped you hard, your mood would almost instantly change. If you jumped into an icy pool, again, your mood and emotions would dramatically change. Hearing is another example. Music can produce profound effects on the state of mind. Calm, soothing music is healing. Loud, raucous music can make one jittery. Yet these emotional events need form and motif in order to cause these changes. The effect of reading musical notes on paper is not the same as that of listening to a great symphony.

Some senses are more powerful than others. The physical sense considered to be the highest is that of smell. Some say that smell is related to memory. For instance, when walking down the street, one can encounter a scent, such as that of baking bread, and almost immediately it reaches the nostrils, one has a flashback to some childhood memory. The science of aromatherapy is based upon the preeminence of the sense of smell. Each flower of nature has its own *rūḥ*, or essence. A pure, natural floral oil may be used for its antiseptic effect on a wound. The Sufis have classified flowers according to their effect upon the soul in its evolution toward God.

Each human being has a *rūḥ*, but not every person's *rūḥ* is the same as the next one's; a sinner is not the same as a saint. Some souls are much more refined than others.

Every person is born into the *maqām an-nafs*, or station of egotism. This is the inevitable first stop in life. The infant is entirely preoccupied with its need for physical satisfaction. It wants food, or to be picked up, and will scream, cry, and spit to make its demands known. It is completely unconcerned about the effects of its own actions. A baby will break an object considered a priceless treasure by an adult, and will laugh about it, at that!

The body in its earliest development cares only to satisfy its animal desires—for food, affection, stimulation of all kinds. Since this is a God-given condition, and a necessary one, infants and children are immune from judgment and punishment. If a small child walks into a supermarket and knocks over a display of bottles, no one says much. Someone cleans it up. But let an adult do it—intentionally, as a child might—and the police may be called.

In the station of egotism, the faculty of reason and judgment has not yet been developed. That comes later on. As a child grows, its parents, or the society at large, generally impress upon it various codes of conduct. In other words, the child learns how to stay on a particular track of behavior. One who deviates from that track will be confronted with various uncomfortable restrictions.

It may be normal and understandable for small children to exist in this state of egotism, but just as they grow out of crawling and regurgitating their food, and develop mature bodies and smooth physical actions, so, too, do we expect that a person's soul will evolve and grow out of egotism.

The Qur'an reveals the proper behavior for conducting this evolutionary progression of the soul. The mode of living spelled out in the Qur'an is called *as-ṣirāṭ al-mustaqīm*: the straight path. For the Sufi, the supreme and sole object of life is to attempt to journey to God, and to do so in the most reasonable and successful manner, and the quickest way as well. Therefore, the straight path is actually a straight line—the shortest distance between two points, which measures the distance between the station of egotism and union with the Beloved, Almighty Allah.

Many people grow into adulthood and even old age without ever departing from this initial stage of egotism, the *maqām an-nafs*. Such people never stop demanding their own way, the endless satisfactions of the body. Taken to the extreme, the whole range of emotional and physical diseases we call chronic and degenerative is a result of remaining in this station too long.

Fearfulness, anxiety, self-doubt, selfishness, insanity, weeping for no reason, depression, paranoia, sexual perversions, and suicide—all are emotional diseases connected with the *maqām an-nafs*, when a person lingers in it into adulthood.

The physical diseases associated with the *maqām an-nafs* can sometimes occur concurrently with the emotional or psychological ones. But for the body, the end result of remaining in the station of egotism includes drug abuse, alcoholism, criminal behavior, obesity, hypoglycemia, blindness and other eye problems, jaundice, heart attack, venereal disease, and cancer. These conditions result from the failure to exercise proper control over one or more of the *nafs* functions, or appetites of the body. Some readers may disagree and say that they know a very nice person who had a heart attack. Understanding the further stations in the evolution of the soul will clarify this matter fully.

The method of escape—or progress—from the station of egotism is to train and discipline the ego and its drives. This means developing willpower, responsibility, consideration, compassion, and courtesy, among other traits. When one succeeds in getting some control over the *nafs* and leaves its stage, one arrives at the *maqām al-qalb*, or station of the heart.

The Arabic word for heart, *qalb*, refers to a wide range of magnificent meanings: heart, mind, soul, understanding, intellect, kernel, marrow, center, the choicest part, core, genuine, pure. Even more interesting is that the word *qalb* also means "permuting," "transmuting," or "turning." For the Sufi, the heart is the means by which all transformation occurs.

Those who occupy the station of the heart have a basic goodness; they feel good about themselves and the world. A person in the *maqām al-qalb* would say, "I want to do only good in the world. I love nature in all its forms. I accept everyone. Oh, what a wonder life is!" Judging by this exalted attitude toward life, one might imagine that no diseases or problems would trouble a person at this stage. The reality is almost the contrary. For persons in the station of the heart are still prone to both emotional and physical imbalances as well as spiritual ones. The emotional and spiritual ailments include the inability to concentrate, forgetfulness, fear of failure, certain types of hypocrisy, excessive emotions such as severe ecstasy, depression, joy, and severe anger, arrogance, and being inconsiderate of others' feelings.

Despite the positive aspects of this station, it is still only the second station of the soul's progress. This stage can be a time of tremendous emotional upheavals, including divorce or other relationship problems, and financial difficulties. This is so because the person feels a surge of ecstasy, a fresh and almost overwhelming excitement toward life. Many who have been involved with the person before he or she ascended to the station of the heart cannot accept the changes they see in their friend. In fact, loss of friends is very common in this stage.

There are also physical problems affiliated with the station of the heart.

While those of the prior state were almost exclusively of a degenerative nature, the diseases and ailments of this stage are chronic and acute. This is so because the body is going through an internal cleansing, a throwing off of toxicity and superfluous matters accumulated in the prior stage. Thus, diseases of the station of the heart include headache (especially migraine), nausea, diarrhea, aches and pains throughout the body, irritability, general toxicity (skin eruptions, scalp problems), fever, and gallbladder and kidney problems.

Whereas the diseases of the station of egotism were severe and often incurable, the conditions of the station of the heart are themselves a kind of self-treatment by the body. Almost all are signs of one or more of the kinds of healing crisis the body undergoes in healing itself. This process may not be pleasant, but it is beneficial.

It is very difficult to continue to the higher stages of soul evolution without a true shaykh. Under his guidance, one may move toward the next stage, *maqām ar-rūḥ* (station of the soul), by following various practices to develop the capacities of mercy, compassion, consideration, and self-discipline to a high pitch of perfection.

No doubt the station of the soul is a blessed state, and anyone occupying it would appear to others as a person of great love and spirituality. But at the same time, there remain physical and emotional imbalances that become part of the mechanism by which the person strives toward God. These conditions deepen faith. The emotional problems of the *maqām ar-rūḥ* include arrogance, pride, self-deception, lack of concentration, giddiness, a frivolous, irreverent attitude to life, and sometimes the habit of degrading others. Note that these are the diseases of this state, not the behavior of one existing in balance in this station. The imbalances may occur when the person has not yet evolved to the point of being entirely immune to the appetites of the *nafs*.

Once, when the great Sufi ᶜAbdul-Qādir Jīlānī (r.a.) was already considered to be a great man of spiritual rank, he was approached by a manifestation that identified itself as Gabriel, the angel of revelation. The manifestation told ᶜAbdul Qadir that he could now dispense with ritual prayer because of his holiness. ᶜAbdul-Qādir recited a verse from the Qur'an which exposed the manifestation as a masquerading *shayṭān* (satan). This demonstrates that the further one travels on the spiritual path, the more certain one may be of insinuations from the devil.

Some of the imbalances of this station are easy to control, some not. One of the more difficult, and offensive, is arrogance. This is the raw, self-referent kind of egotism that leads a person to say, "I am better than others. I pray all day. I fast. I meditate, and look at all these garbage people in the world. They're sinners!" This may be the truth in some form about certain people, but it is an injury to them, and it mars one's own spiritual development to express it. It must be appreciated that each person has evolved to a particular point by the decision of Almighty God. No matter how sunk into the life of the world people may be, they still have within them the spark of divinity. They also can advance, and it is the duty of a truly spiritual person not to condemn them, but to befriend them so that they might be led out of their misery and onto the right path of living.

Some physical problems are associated with the station of the soul. These include auto-intoxication (from excessive breathing practices), various kinds of nervous tremors, fatigue, corrupted appetite, and fever.

There are two forms of fever. The first, occurring in the stations of egotism and the heart, is an intense heat developed by the body to refine and process out superfluous toxic matters. The second kind of fever, occurring in the later stations, constitutes a deep spiritual cleansing, causing, as the Prophet Muhammad (s.a.w.s.) has said, "the sins to fall off like leaves being shed from a tree." These fevers burn off impurities on the soul level. Even some of the prophets were subject to frequent fevers. The holy people who experience fever at this level are not being corrected for vile living habits. As one Sufi said, "In the beginning you repent for wrong actions and sins; at the end, you repent for forgetting God even for a second." It is this latter condition that is being treated in the station of the soul.

It can happen that persons in the station of the soul skid off into lunatic behavior, especially if they have no guide. They may fall into the most destructive kinds of self-illusion. One can never rest at any stage or assume that one will never fall back.

When it comes to a spiritual physician or Sufi treating a person for a disease, it now becomes clear that the saint and the person dwelling in the station of egotism would require drastically different modes of treatment—even though they both may report fever as the main symptom.

The question may arise whether a person may overlap from one station into the next. This does not occur. A station is a resting place. As such, once one enters a station, one will remain until death or until retreating or advancing into another station. There are, however, innumerable immediate conditions occurring in each station, and these conditions are called *ḥāl*. Literally, *ḥāl* means "change." It is linked by sound to *ḥall*, meaning an untying or unloosing, a dissolving. In this sense, it means when we lose our senses, such is the extreme fervor of the Sufis during their recitations of *dhikr*, when it is not uncommon to see one of the members fall senseless to the ground, having glimpsed something of *ḥaqīqah* (truth) or *maʿrifah* (ecstasy).

The fourth station is the *maqām as-sirr*, the station of divine secrets. The word *sirr* (pl. *asrār*) refers to the greatest mystery, which cannot be imagined, and even when experienced, it cannot be believed. The word also has other meanings: coition, the middle or best part of anything, richest land, root, origin, and tomb.

This is the station referred to by Allah when He said, "There are certain of my servants who cease not seeking nearness to me by means of voluntary worship, until I become the lips with which they speak, the eyes with which they see, the ears by which they hear, the hand wherewith they hold, and the foot by which they step." The fortunate ones in the station of divine secrets can understand the mechanisms by which the whole universe is held in place. They have fully developed powers of clairaudience and can read the thoughts of others. Angels come to them with information from the unseen realms.

One day someone asked the Prophet Muhammad (ṣ.a.w.s.), "What was all of this universe created for? How does it exist?" The Prophet answered, "I don't know the answer. I'll have to go ask the angel Gabriel." So he went and asked Gabriel, who answered, "I don't know the answer to that, I'll have to go ask Allah." So Gabriel asked Allah, then returned and said, "Allah said, 'I have created the skies and heavens simply as a beautiful sight and an entertainment for you, and to create wonder and awe of My majesty and power. I want the blinking stars to uplift and delight you and cause you to marvel at My creation.'" When Allah was asked how He did all of this, Gabriel reported that He said, "I did not create humans with the mental capacity to comprehend the means and mechanisms by which I have done this. Even if I told you, you would not understand. But at the instant of death, when the veils are torn away, you will immediately see how it is done, and you will be astonished at My ingenuity. I am the best of creators. As complicated and complex as I have made the heavens, I have made the human body infinitely more complex." The Prophet Muhammad (s.a.w.s.), who most certainly existed in the highest of stations, was able to receive this kind of information. The average person would never attain to this exalted state and favor of the Almighty God.

The persons admitted to the station of divine secrets have passed the most excruciating tests and are no longer seeking any egotistical aspect of human life. They do not desire fame, wealth, or exciting sensations. They exist only for and by virtue of a very exclusive and intimate relationship with the Creator and the celestial population. Nonetheless, they are still human, and some physical and emotional events do occur on this plane as well. It is not correct to call these events "diseases," really; they are rather imbalances or sidetracks that can cause one to descend from this state or to languish in this station and not continue further, to reach the goal of Allah. The primary imbalances of the station of divine secrets include false interpretation of divine phenomena, irrationality, lack of interest in earthly life, incoherent babbling, heart pain, and heart burning.

At this point, it should be explained that a person in one station generally cannot leap several stations ahead or above. A young child may be able to ride a bicycle well, but certainly could not pilot a supersonic jet. This is not to demean the child or glorify the pilot. But a person who has attained a particular station can function in and understand any of the lower stations—just as the pilot, having ridden a bicycle as a child, could continue to do so as an adult.

The self-deception referred to in this station of divine secrets would be a condition of this *maqām*. But a *ḥāl* would be the mode in which this self-deception manifests itself. Not everyone in this or any other station would experience all of the *ḥāl*s that could occur in that station.

The physical events that occur in the *maqām as-sirr* are fever, a sense of difficulty in breathing, and sometimes a sense of suffocating. These particular afflictions occur because arrival at this stage requires years of breathing practices. Imbalances can occur if these practices are done incorrectly or excessively. Moreover, it is not uncommon at this stage that one is bothered by events of the nonmanifest realms. Interference from jinns is an example (although they can bother people at any stage, even infants). Or one may be carrying on certain kinds of relations with disembodied souls and become affected by this interchange. In these cases, various kinds of spiritual practices involving breathing would be employed as remedies.

For the Sufis, the main source of breathing practices is the Holy Qur'an itself. The various breath starts and stops are marked in the text of the Qur'an and employ degrees of difficulty up through eleven levels of recitation. The vowels, in particular, are frequently elongated and held for more than a normal single beat in reciting. Although only a few persons as a practical matter can recite at the advanced levels, it is possible to find cassette tapes of such performances by shaykhs reciting the Holy Qur'an. In these phenomenally stirring recordings, one can hear sustained recitations lasting up to two minutes with one breath expulsion, and movement through four and five octave ranges.

Beyond the station of divine secrets is the *maqām al-qurb*. The definition of *qurb* is "nearness," but it also connotes drawing near, approach, neighborhood, relationship, and kinship. One in this station indeed enjoys the view of the neighborhood of the Most High—that is, the highest heaven, containing the *ʿarsh*, or Throne of the Almighty. One occupying the status of this station has a vantage of this created world, but also glimpses into the next world, the world of other created forms.

At this stage there are very few imbalances or difficulties, strictly in terms of health and disease, but those that do exist can be very severe. One of the conditions is excessive ecstasy. A person affected with this condition is called *majdhūb*. Such people lose virtually all interest in or connection with the world. They are in a state of joy at all times and do not care whether they sleep, eat, or are clothed. They are divinely intoxicated and absorbed in the Beloved.

I met such a man once living out in the pastoral countryside near Paghman, Afghanistan. He was said by his followers to be about 125 years old. As I and my companions entered the high-walled garden of his compound, we saw a small man sitting hunched over rows of potted geraniums. From time to time, he would pick a few bright red blossoms and eat them. He shared these treats with squirrels and other small animals that scurried around him without fear. Later, upstairs in his room, he behaved in a manner that would alarm anyone uninformed about this station. He never spoke clearly or directly, but one could catch snatches of his conversations addressed to the inhabitants of the angelic realms. Birds flew in and out of the open windows. As we were leaving, he offered one of my companions a "gift," which he held out like a treasure in his cupped palms. The gift turned out to be a dirt-smeared, half-eaten peach pit! Such is the condition of those in the station of nearness, who perceive reality on an entirely other plane. This state is interesting and beautiful in its way, but it is not the goal. In fact, most shaykhs are of the opinion that it is an inferior and undesirable condition.

Some people in this station do not speak. Cases are recorded of some who went for over twenty years without speaking, being so overwhelmed that they had no desire or ability to communicate. Other difficulties include forgetfulness and genuine insanity. The person forgets from one moment to the next what he is saying or doing. Some of the practices—involving both breath and mental contemplation—are so profound and intense that the person may lose his mind entirely. This is rare, however.

Remarkable similarities may be observed between the conditions occurring in these latter stages of spiritual evolution and the behavior of the mentally ill. In the East, many people on the street exhibit such bizarre behavior that they would immediately be locked up if they did the same thing in the West. Yet a true diagnosis of their condition would require a consideration of the imbalances of the soul.

A problem not mentioned yet but common to all of the stations (and yet more of a danger in the station of nearness than any other) is that of attributing divinity to oneself, God protect us from such a thing. And, although it is painful to even think of it, a related imbalance—the most severe—is disbelief in God.

The higher and further one rises in the evolution of the soul, the more one is tested. People at this level have long since extinguished their carnal desires and egotistic traits. But they frequently are very successful in leading others to the path of truth and righteousness, and therefore are constantly being bothered by all of the malevolent forces—*shayaṭin* (devils), jinns, *dayo paree* (ghosts), and similar troublemakers.

I have heard people say that they themselves listen to God, or that they have received guidance directly from God. They ought to recall that the only means Allah has ever used to relate to humans is the angel Gabriel (with the sole exception of Moses, once). There are many warnings about assuming oneself to be adequate armor against the delusions of the evil ones, both human and nonhuman. The great shaykh Junayd (r.a.) said, "He who takes himself as a teacher has taken Satan as his guide."

One more station exists, and the Sufis call it *maqām al-wiṣāl*, or union with Allah. Here God is your Beloved and you are the lover, and you are wedded together in Divine Unity for all time. This station, unlike all of those which precede it, cannot be attained by effort. Almighty Allah makes the decision and chooses whom He will.

The tradition relating the manner of selection for this station is moving. It is quoted from the Holy Prophet Muhammad (s.a.w.s.) on the authority of Hazrat Ibn Masᶜūd (r.a.):

> Among the creatures of Allah, there are three hundred people who bear a special relationship with Allah and whose hearts are similar to that of the prophet Adam, peace be upon him. And forty whose hearts are similar to that of the prophet Moses, peace be upon him. Seven are those whose hearts are similar to that of the prophet Abraham, peace be upon him. Five are those whose hearts are similar to that of the archangel Gabriel. Three are those whose hearts are like that of the angel Michael. There is one servant among the creatures of Allah the Almighty whose heart is like the angel Isrāfīl. When one servant dies, Allah chooses one from among the three to replace him. When one among the three dies, one from among the five is admitted to his place. When one among the five dies, one from among the seven is admitted in his place. When any of the seven dies, one from among the forty is admitted to his place. When any one of the forty dies, one from among the three hundred is admitted to his place. When one from among the three hundred dies, one from among the people in general is admitted. So, because of them, Allah the Almighty administers life, death, rainfall, creation, and rids humanity of misfortunes.

All of the three hundred persons would be characteristically smiling at all times and would have no concerns whatsoever of the world. They do not need to eat, drink, or sleep. They have transcended human bounds and can soar—literally—anywhere they like, on earth and through the heavens. Only a few in human history have come to this status. It is impossible to describe in words. It is the real goal of existence and involves the promise we each made to our Creator before we came into this life.

These people are termed *walī* (pl. *awliyā'*), meaning "beloved friends of God." They are the real vicegerents of God on earth. Generally, they are not known to the world at large. The *awliyā'* are informed about and have access to the mechanisms to control and affect all human events, and it is they whom Allah uses to unfold the divine plan on earth. The means they use are with the knowledge of Allah.

Only one who has attained admittance among the three hundred or the lesser numbers is properly termed a Sufi. All others are rather aspirants to Sufism.

By the time one attains the station of proximity there are no physical ailments left. The only physical event remaining is the mode by which one will die. Usually, people at this station do not die from disease as such, but rather they are informed by the Angel of Death of the precise time for their departure, and so can make preparations for it. My shaykh wrote me the exact date of his death one month before it occurred. He worked, fully alert, up until the morning of his passing. Then, at two P.M., he lay down and began reciting the profession of faith (*Lā ilāha illā LLāh, Muḥammadun rasūlu Llāh*) until he expired, just after sunset (which happened on the birthday of the Prophet, s.a.w.s.). *Mā shā' Allāh.*

For such persons, when they pass out of human life, it is a blessed event, even a celebration, for they have long since given up relating to the world with their bodies. Instead, they have soared high into the spiritual realms with their souls and are able to traverse not only this but the other universes as well. No one can disturb or contradict them. Even the most determined criminals or violent armies would be powerless against the Sufi. Such persons are immune from the difficulties of the world.

Generally, one is not accepted into the circles of shaykhs until one has attained the station of the soul or higher. This acceptance by the aspirant of the duties imposed upon the shaykhs is formalized in a special ceremony of initiation, called *bayʿat* (pledge). The founder of the Chishti Order in India, Hazrat Khwāja Muʿīnuddīn (r.a.), has offered an account of his own initiation at the hands of his shaykh, ʿUthmān Harūnī (r.a.).This ceremony transpired in the year A.H. 561, after Khwāja Muʿīnuddīn had spent a full twenty years in training and service with his shaykh. The great saint described his *bayʿat* thus:

> I had the honor of appearing before my shaykh, Hazrat ʿUthmān, in the presence of many other spiritual luminaries. I bowed my head in solemn reverence. Hazrat ʿUthmān asked me to offer two *rakʿat*s of *ṣalāt*. I did it. He then directed me to face the Kaʿbah at Mecca. I did it. He then asked me to recite the Qur'anic chapter Sūrat al-Baqarah. I did it. He told me to repeat praise and blessings for the Holy Prophet (s.a.w.s.) and his family (a.s.) twenty-one times and to say *Subḥān Allāh* sixty times. I did it.
>
> After that, he stood up, took my hands in his own, and looked toward the heavens, saying, "Let me present you to Allah." After that he cut off my hair with a scissors and then put a special cap [*kolah chahar tarki*] on my head and asked me to sit down. He then asked me to repeat Sūrat al-Ikhlāṣ one thousand times. I did it. He then said, "Among our followers there is only one day and one night's probation [*mujāhadah*], hence go and do it today." Accordingly I spent the whole of one day and one night in continuous *ṣalāt* and reappeared before him.
>
> He asked me to sit down and repeat Sūrat al-Ikhlāṣ again one thousand times. I did so. He then instructed me, "Look toward the heavens." When I raised my eyes toward the heavens, he inquired, "How far do you see?" I

said, "Up to *al-ᶜarsh al-muᶜalā*" [the Zenith of the Divine Throne]. He then said, "Look below." I did so. He inquired again, "How far do you see?" I said, "Down to the *taḥtath-tharā*" [the Abyss of Hell].

He then asked me to sit down and repeat Surat al-Ikhlāṣ one thousand times. I did it. He then told me, "Look toward the heavens." When I did so, he inquired, "How far do you see now?" I said, "Up to the *ᶜaẓmat*" (the Dazzlement of God's Glory). He then told me, "Close your eyes." I did so, and after a moment, he told me, "Open your eyes." I did so. He then held up the first two fingers of his right hand and inquired, "What do you see through them?" I said, "I see the eighteen thousand worlds." When he heard this he said, "Now your work is over." He then looked toward a brick lying nearby and asked me to pick it up. When I did so, I found some gold coins under it. He asked me to go and distribute them among the poor and the needy, which I did. He then instructed me to remain with him for some time.

Thus with obedience and the grace of Allah does the soul progress from its state at inception—of helpless egotism—to the divine unity, if Allah wills it.

The means of passing from lower to higher stations is by opposing and controlling the appetites of the *nafs*. And in this endeavor, the Sufis have received special practices that are designed by Allah Himself to produce the most sure, rapid, and profound results.

Failure often overwhelms people who desire, or think they desire, to take up and maintain a spiritual orientation to life. This is so because the ego is the greatest test there is. We may wake up any morning with the firmest resolve that we will concentrate only on the purest, most blessed, and highest thoughts. Yet all it takes is a phone call, telling us that we are overdrawn at the bank, or that the children have broken a window, and before we know what has happened, we have lost our concentration. Only later in the afternoon do we recall our resolution to remember God.

Therefore, one must constantly restate and restart one's intention all the time. At first, it may be difficult, and failures may occur. But sooner than one would imagine, the intention leads to a habit, the most positive habit possible. After a time, you don't forget.

Gradually the aspirant lets go of worldly ambitions and concentrates solely on the spiritual goals. In India at the headquarters of our Chishti Order, there is the resting place of our *murshid*, Hazrat Khwāja Muᶜīnuddīn Chishtī (r.a.). Beneath the shrine—the *dargah*—are about one hundred small cells (*hujrahs*), which are assigned to shaykhs of the order for use during visits to Ajmer. These cells exist for the performance of the *chilla*, a forty-day-and-night seclusion, underground and in darkness, with a minimum of food and water. This practice constitutes a kind of rehearsal for being in the grave. The Sufis, realizing the inevitable nature of death, take the opportunity while still living to see what the grave is like, and prepare for this extended time of seclusion. While in this seclusion for forty days and nights, one is under the direction of one's shaykh, who prescribes certain recitations and practices, which serve to extinguish the fires of the *nafs* and annul the lower desires. One cannot undergo this ritual alone or according to one's own thinking. The dangers are awesome. This is only one of the important reasons one needs a living master to guide one at all times.

If we read the testimony of all of the greatest people who lived—the prophets (a.s.)—we find that they were the most fearful of what awaited them in the grave and in the next life. These people were the most humble, most righteous and selfless people who lived; and they all were constantly aware of their shortcomings and worried about their ultimate fate before their Lord. How much more ought ordinary people to express such concern.

The foregoing descriptions of the stations of the soul's evolution are of necessity greatly simplified, and many decades are required under true teachers and optimum circumstances to achieve meaningful results. There are schools that teach a person how to fix an automobile engine, which require two or three years just to learn the basics. How much more time and complexity are involved in learning how to fix the harsh workings of a disordered soul.

There is a difference between a serious seeker who comes before a shaykh to find the anchor for life and the person who *is* the guide. The difference between these two persons—seeker and sought, disciple and master, *murīd* and *shaykh*—is that the shaykh gives and the student receives. The student comes asking, seeking, demanding—still in need. The transition occurs when one no longer remains crying for breast milk, for the teacher's aid and attention, but instead becomes one who demands to give. And no one can stop the giving. It is like going through the midpoint of an hourglass. One who has passed through that small and difficult stricture may not be a teacher yet, but at least is looking out to the other side.

It's like being a river rushing down the side of a mountain, trying to reach the ocean. When the ocean is reached, there is a great, tranquil merging, a new existence. What need is there then to be a little river, noisily running over the rocks? There are no more barriers when one has reached the ocean of divine mercy.

So those who arrive at the final destination—union with Allah—are of the chosen ones, the Sufis. Their status in the eyes of Allah is one of great favor, but below that of the prophets (peace be upon them all). They are not prophets, nor have they ever claimed such a thing for themselves. However, they stand as a testament and inspiration to the heights that human beings may achieve, by sincerely following the advice and loving guidance of the Great, the Praised, the Glorious, the Holy, the Lord of Angels and the Spirit, the Exalted, the Glorified Allah the Almighty. *Al-ḥāmdu li-Lāhi rabb il-ᶜālamīn!*

Now let us turn to the health aspects of the body, the mind, and the soul, and take notice of the modes of treatment employed by the Sufis in treating various imbalances to restore people to full health.

4

Food and Health

The stomach is the home of disease.
Diet is the main medicine.

Prophet Muhammad (s.a.w.s.)
Saḥīḥ Muslim

The worldly life is one of the stages of the journey to God, and the body is the vehicle for this journey. As such, it behooves the traveler to maintain the body in optimum condition, so that the diversions of discomfort and pain do not distract one from concentration upon the goal.

Digestion is the process of taking in nutrients through the mouth and then refining those elements in the body. When it is said that the stomach is the home of disease, this means that disease arises when this digestive process becomes unbalanced. "Diet is the main medicine" is taken to mean that we should first use foods themselves to rebalance and rebuild the digestive process. The foods are used as vehicles for conveying certain healing formulas—both herbal and nonphysical—to the body.

The possible exception to this general rule occurs when the body and its organs have been damaged so severely that there remains no regenerative power to rebuild an organ or bodily system. In such cases, surgery or other radical modes might be the treatment of choice. However, if the principles of health are followed throughout life, from earliest childhood onward, one need have no more fear of falling ill than being struck by lightning. Indeed, I have known quite a few men and women (mainly residing in the East) who have never had a day of illness in their lives. They had never had so much as a headache and never visited a doctor or a hospital. Perhaps health is best defined as that state in which one never need be aware of the body. In other words, a healthy person receives no signals of pain, disturbance, or discomfort—all of which signify some kind of imbalance in the body. Nonetheless, if we recall the pathways of the soul's evolution, originating in the station of egotism, we know that these imbalances have developed in many people.

Let us review the process of digestion so as to determine how and why imbalances occur.

One characteristic of Sufi shaykhs that seems to predominate over all others is that they are extremely hospitable and capable of offering some of the most delicious and satisfying meals imaginable. Many stories about the shaykhs revolve around some aspect of food, not only intake, but also abstinence.

Once I was visiting near Balkh, Afghanistan, and wanted to go and sit with a shaykh I had heard of, a descendant of Hazrat Mawlānā Rūmī (r.a.). The *imam* (prayer leader) of the main mosque at Balkh gave me directions to the old shaykh's *khanaqah* (compound), in the village of Esrak, about fifteen kilometers from Balkh. After a most interesting journey to the village, I found the shaykh standing in the doorway, as though he had been expecting me. Once inside, I saw a group of old dervishes sitting huddled in a circle, about to commence the noon meal. The shaykh invited me to join them, and I sat down. In a few minutes a large wooden bowl was brought and placed before the shaykh. There was one wooden spoon in the bowl. The shaykh took a portion for himself, replaced the spoon, and handed the serving bowl to the man seated on his right. After a half-dozen men had their turns, the bowl came to me. I took a spoonful of a cucumber and yogurt soup, which was unbelievably delicious, despite its simplicity. In all my memories, I cannot recall any meal being better than that soup shared with a handful of dervishes perched atop the world.

One of the great Chishti shaykhs, Hazrat Niẓāmuddīn Awliyā' (r.a.), kept a half-dozen of his *murīd*s with him for more than seven years, and all the while prevented them from eating to their fill. Frequently they were on the edge of starvation. One day a disheveled beggar arrived at the door and broke an earthen bowl of flour before the eyes of the starving dervishes. From that day forth, Hazrat Niẓāmuddīn provided the most magnificent feasts for the whole city of Delhi up till the end of his life.

Why are shaykhs so involved in providing food to their followers? First of all, it is a good service to feed the hungry, if they are genuinely in need. But even more important, the shaykhs have a certain knowledge of the effects of food on the body and the stages of the soul's evolution, and so they can frequently benefit the students and the sick by the choice of foods served at meals.

The serving of food must be conceived of on the broadest possible scale. By this I mean that the person preparing and serving the food—be it mother, father, servant, or shaykh—must take into account all of the factors relevant to the season or time of year, the time of day, the climate, altitude, distance from the sea, any prevalent diseases or viruses, unusual migration of insects, and so forth. People who live close to nature are able to observe all of these factors and many others as well.

The conception and intention brought to the preparation of a meal are the most important things that bear on food. In the United States, it seems that not only do people seldom consciously think about food in this way, but they really do not even take the time to sit down and eat properly, preferring to have a paper-wrapped clod slapped into their hands as they drive by a window.

In my family, my wife, Iman, and I are constantly conferring with each other about what foods ought to be included in the menu. She'll inform me what small things are going on with our children's health, or what particular foods are coming onto the market by season. We make adjustments according to the situation. For example, it is a very common notion in the East that milk and fish should never be consumed together. Biochemical research has shown that milk and fish both have a high concentration of a particular amino acid. When they are eaten together, the concentration is so great that it may cause allergic reactions.

Another important consideration is that fruits and vegetables at the beginning of the growing season have a healing quality, while those at the end of the growing season can produce disease. This is confirmed with apples, for example, which are very tart and astringent early in the growing season. But after the freeze, the sugar content soars and can easily cause excessive mucus buildup. Flus, colds, and the like may result.

Attention must be given to the selection and buying of foods. Where are you going to buy your food products? Where do they come from? Are they treated with chemicals? If so, what chemicals? Most foods should be obtained from the locale in which you reside. Always buy onions and potatoes grown locally (or within one day's journey), because they contain the cure and antidote for all of the little viruses, bugs, and special bacterial strains that occur in your region. One should not forgo onions from one's own neighborhood in favor of those trucked in from a thousand miles away. Of course, if you live in an area where potatoes and onions are not grown at all, then you generally should not eat those particular foods. Eskimos seldom, if ever, eat bananas!

People who enter a supermarket are often pleased by the sight of the bonanza of foods, a virtual cornucopia. Yet almost all of the foods, including fresh fruits and vegetables, have been severely altered with chemical additives and treatments. It may be marvelous that you can obtain Egyptian mangoes, Bolivian pomegranates, and Mexican bananas at your corner grocery, but that does not necessarily mean they will sustain you properly.

Conventional advice about food selection emphasizes consuming the main food groups daily. Some people refine the concept somewhat and suggest choosing whole grains, fresh fruits and vegetables in season, and so forth. Others offer analysis of the vitamin, mineral, and nutrient content of the foods as the key to eating for health. The Sufis view the matter somewhat differently. Just as they perceive the soul or essence of the body as the most important, so, too, do they seek the essence of food as the most important element.

Let us assume for the moment that we have selected the correct foods and have the best intentions in regard to feeding our family and friends. The next stage is the actual cooking of the food. I have said many times that the most important hospital in the world is your own kitchen, because it is here that the essence of the food is extracted, and health gained or lost.

If the food is being prepared correctly—taking sufficient time for each stage—the first thing that occurs in the kitchen is the most delightful explosions of scents. When onions are heated in olive oil, for example, the volatile oils and essence are driven off into the air. When you add spices such as cinnamon, ginger, cardamom, and similar aromatic spices, anyone who comes into the house and gets a whiff of these wonderful scents is immediately uplifted.

The matter of scents is important, and indeed many today are becoming interested in the essences of floral substances (including what we generally call spices) and their effect on health. The body responds to all of these smells in various ways. As the nose perceives certain odors of cooking, information is delivered to the internal organs that a meal is being readied. The stomach, gallbladder, liver, colon, thyroid gland, and other endocrine glands—all respond in their own ways. Moreover, the essences of oils, driven off by the heating, can themselves alter the temperament of internal organs and thus affect health greatly. At the very least, cooking fragrances are responsible for altering the body to conclude the prior meal's digestion. When people come into the dining room only moments before eating, and thus are deprived of the intake of scents prior to the meal (or even throughout the day), some of the most important initial stages of digestion are lost. In fact, the process of digestion actually begins at the time of the mental conception of a meal.

These scented vapors not only affect the bodily functions, including the skin, but also have a beneficial influence on the eyes. Onions, which make you cry when you cut them, are the best example of this. Many injurious toxins are built up as a normal result of the thinking and emotional life. Particularly since many people think that crying is somehow unmanly or weak, the tendency to release superfluous matters through the eyes by crying is suppressed. During cooking, the vapors of onions as well as other spices encourage elimination through the eyes. When onions are cut in the kitchen, it is surely not a mournful matter.

When I cook, I start at noon. To me, preparing meals for others is one of the most enjoyable and wonderful things a human can do. Cooking is healing in its essence. I have one dish made of basmati rice with chopped pistachios, almonds, raisins, and tiny carrots slivered into pieces the size and shape of toothpicks. I need about three dozen large carrots to make this dish for eight or ten people. I always sit down with a sharp knife and spend an hour or more at this task of slicing, until a huge pile of carrot slivers is sitting before me.

One day someone helping in the kitchen saw me doing this and informed me, "I have a great idea. Here, put those carrots in the food processor, and the job will be done in less than a minute!" I thanked my assistant for the suggestion and then explained that the reason I preferred doing the job by hand was that with each slice I made a little prayer that the food be a healing influence for the person who eats it. So the thought of desiring wellness for people also needs to be added to the foods that you prepare for them.

We certainly can tell the difference between food eaten in a restaurant and food prepared properly in the home. Too often, the people who work in public eating establishments have no concern whatsoever for the food they serve (food which almost always is prepared by machines). In fact, many people having jobs in restaurants are angry and disgusted that they have to work there in the first place. The mental vibrations of such people inevitably work their way into the food.

Let us now assume that we have the best food, prepared according to the correct methods, and are ready to put it into our mouths. Even before we put the food into the mouth, we have to think for a second: Where does this food come from, and what is our purpose in consuming it? For the Sufi, the eating of food is a time of fellowship, a celebration of life, and a rededication of life to the highest ideals of human existence. Before eating, the Sufi says, "*Bismi Llāhi ir-Raḥmān, ir-Raḥīm*: In the name of God, the most merciful, the most compassionate. O my Lord! I will eat this food only to be a better servant of yours. Use this food to uplift me and uplift all of your humanity. *Āmīn*."

The reason for eating is not simply to derive pleasure. It is to maintain the body, which is the vehicle for conveyance of the soul and the means by which we improve and give strength and gracefulness to the soul. Only after applying such an invocation to the food do we put it into our mouths, *in shā' Allāh*.

The refinement, or digestion, of food requires from one to eight hours, depending upon the food. Science has delved into the biochemical structures of foods and the body and derived some facts and theories that purport to explain what goes on during digestion.

The most important concept relating to human physical health is centered on the notions conveyed by two Persian words, *sardi* and *garmi*, meaning "hot" and "cold." Before explaining this concept fully, let me say that the entire process of digestion should be thought of as one of heating, or cooking, the nutrient substances. There is a Persian word, *pokhta*, which means "cooking," but also refers to what the body does in breaking down food into its composite nutrients. *Pokhta* means that something is cooked and ready to serve. For example, one knows that a curry is *pokhta* when the ghee or oil is floating lightly, shimmering and glittering, on top of the sauce. Until then, it is not ready to serve, is not fully cooked.

There is a moment of ripeness to everything. We can easily see when a fruit is unripe, and we would not eat it until it is ripe. The gross cooking of food leads to a moment of ripeness, and the body itself "cooks" the food down until it is also ripened and ready to assimilate into the blood or tissues or enter into other chemical interactions.

In other words, something is ripe when it is at the optimum moment of growth or refinement. In the processing of foods by the body, a series of digestions occur, beginning with the action of enzymes in the mouth. This action creates heat, slight though it may be. To this heat is added the heat of friction, caused by the grinding of the food by the teeth. After the food is swallowed into the stomach, another cooking occurs—the heat of hydrochloric acid. Each of these heatings changes the nature of the food. If one lacks the proper levels of enzymes in the mouth, or fails to chew the food sufficiently, or if there is a hydrochloric acid deficiency, then digestion will be impaired from the start.

When the digestion in the stomach is finished, the food is a semifluid mass called chyme. Exiting from the stomach, the chyme travels through the small intestine, where further enzymes act upon it. Then it arrives at the site of the liver.

Eastern and Western medicine have taken virtually irreconcilable views of digestion from this point onward. Western science tries to identify each components of the nutrient—vitamins, amino acids, enzymes, caloric values, proteins, fats, and so forth. Eastern medicine feels such an effort is by and large useless. This is so because each liver cell contains more than one thousand enzymes. Or it should be said rather that Western pathologists have acknowledged that more than a thousand enzymes exist in each liver cell, of which they know specifically how only about two dozen actually work in the body! In fact, there may be billions of enzymes in each liver cell. This is not known or unknown as yet. In any case, to base one's theories on somewhat less than three percent of the total possibilities is to rely on mere guesswork.

Eastern medicine takes a much more interesting view of the digestive process—a view that can be understood by anyone, even young children, and that provides the basic framework for the selection of foods to maintain or regain health quickly and easily. These concepts are consistent with all systems of medicine in the world—Chinese, Ayurvedic, Hippocratic, Galenic, Arabic, and Hebraic. In other words, all of the medical and health systems of the world have agreed with these concepts for thousands of years—except Western biochemical medicine.

The key to healthful eating habits is in understanding two notions: the four bodily essences, and the heating and cooling effects of foods. These concepts are so important to human health that the next chapter is devoted to them.

5

Akhlāṭ: The Four Essences of the Body

The four essences of the physical body arise at the site of the liver and are part of the process of digestion. Each of these essences, or *akhlāṭ* (sing. *khilṭ*), is produced as the food is broken down into ever-smaller components of nutrients and by-products. The accompanying chart summarizes the origin and fate of each of the four essences.

Let us now focus upon the four essences:

Blood Essence: Hot and Moist
Phlegm Essence: Cold and Moist
Bilious Essence: Hot and Dry
Atrabilious Essence: Cold and Dry

Each of these essences has a characteristic temperament of heat and moisture associated with it. When this temperament is altered or disturbed, imbalance occurs, frequently leading to one or more disease conditions. (I use the term "intemperament" for such imbalances.) Like the other essences described in Sufi healing, the *akhlāṭ* do not exist as separate entities, but only as a part of the entire process of digestion. When the body no longer functions, the essences also cease to exist.

To illustrate how these essences function, let us consider in some detail the phlegm essence.

The phlegm essence comes into being as part of the third stage of digestion, and is formed from the less choice nutrient parts (the choicer parts having already been utilized in the formation of blood and its essence). Phlegm is used in many ways in the body: as a lubricant, as a shield against foreign matter, including bacteria, and as a coating of the internal viscera, among other things. Phlegm by nature is somewhat sticky, but it frequently can be observed to change its character—to salty, thin, rough, watery, and so forth. Normal phlegm will always be the result of a cold and moist essence. When the essence moves to either a hotter or colder degree, the phlegm itself is altered. Sometimes this alteration is necessary as part of the healing process.

The *ḥakīms*, physicians of the physical diseases, have worked out a codified system that categorizes all diseases arising from disturbances of this third stage of digestion by the nature of the phlegm. Likewise, all of the other essences can alter and produce imbalances, and specific symptoms are associated with a particular imbalance of each essence. It follows, then, that the first course of treatment is to *restore the essence to its natural balance*.

Now, it is rather easy to arrive at a diagnosis, by first determining which stage of digestion is affected and then looking for the signs of excess heat or moisture (or its opposite). Although four factors are associated with each essence—heat, cold, moisture, dryness—these can be reduced to two, heat and cold (*garmi* and *sardi* in Persian), because moisture is a function of heat, which drives off moisture.*

Of course, the diagnosis of a complicated imbalance belongs in the realm of an expert physician. However, there exists a complete system of dietetics according to the foregoing principles and essences. This system of food selection is based upon the two factors of heat and cold.

When we say that a food is hot, we do not mean that it is actually hot to the taste, nor do we refer to its caloric value. Rather, a hot food is one that creates a net effect in the body which promotes metabolism. A food that is cold in its essence has a net effect of lowering metabolism. In other words, if we had a thermometer that measured temperature in billionths of degrees rather than tenths, we could observe a slight increase in body temperature whenever a hot food was consumed. And the reverse would be true of eating a cold food: The temperature would drop slightly.

The single most important factor in this dietetic system is that foods contain sufficient metabolic heat to allow digestion to be completed. As the Prophet Muhammad (s.a.w.s.) has said, "The main cause of disease is eating one meal on top of another." This means that the food first consumed is not fully digested and assimilated before a new meal is taken. Of course if one eats every twenty minutes, such a condition would occur. But what is meant here is that the food is not fully digested owing to lack of metabolic heat. This notion becomes clearer when we look at the metabolic values of many common foods, given in the accompanying chart (page 48).

Although it is beyond the scope of this book to present the entire system of medicine (known as Ṭibb) that has evolved from these marvelous prin-

*The prince of physicians, Ḥakīm Abū ʿAlī ibn Sīnā, known as Avicenna in the West, wrote an eighteen-volume encyclopedia of medicine, in which can be found a complete discussion of the essences and which diseases result from which imbalance of each. I have published a book, translated from Persian sources including the works of Avicenna, which introduces this system of physical medicine for the lay public and natural practitioners: *Natural Medicine* (London: Wildwood House, 1980).

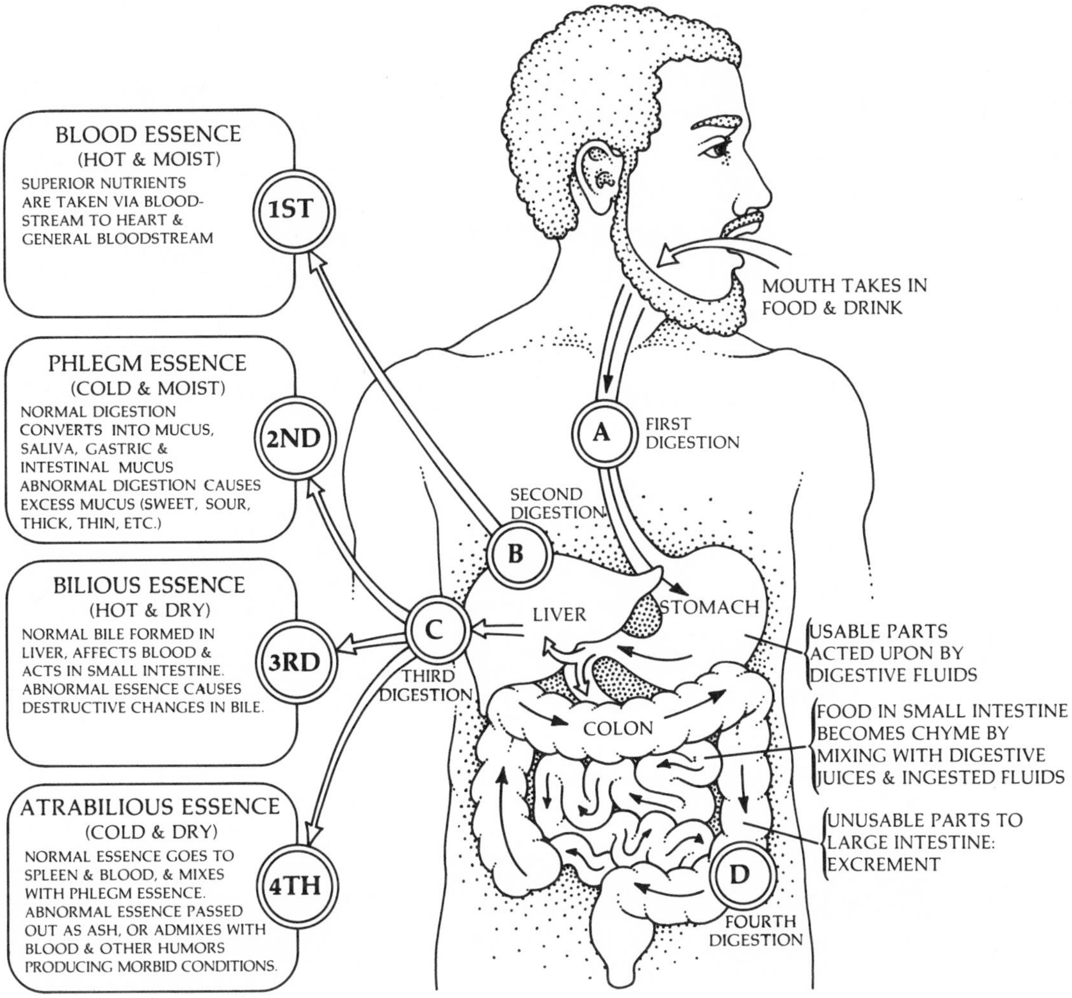

BLOOD ESSENCE
(HOT & MOIST)
SUPERIOR NUTRIENTS ARE TAKEN VIA BLOOD-STREAM TO HEART & GENERAL BLOODSTREAM
1ST
PHLEGM ESSENCE
(COLD & MOIST)
NORMAL DIGESTION CONVERTS INTO MUCUS, SALIVA, GASTRIC & INTESTINAL MUCUS
ABNORMAL DIGESTION CAUSES EXCESS MUCUS (SWEET, SOUR, THICK, THIN, ETC.)
2ND
BILIOUS ESSENCE
(HOT & DRY)
NORMAL BILE FORMED IN LIVER, AFFECTS BLOOD & ACTS IN SMALL INTESTINE.
ABNORMAL ESSENCE CAUSES DESTRUCTIVE CHANGES IN BILE.
3RD
ATRABILIOUS ESSENCE
(COLD & DRY)
NORMAL ESSENCE GOES TO SPLEEN & BLOOD, & MIXES WITH PHLEGM ESSENCE.
ABNORMAL ESSENCE PASSED OUT AS ASH, OR ADMIXES WITH BLOOD & OTHER HUMORS PRODUCING MORBID CONDITIONS.
4TH
MOUTH TAKES IN FOOD & DRINK
A
FIRST DIGESTION
SECOND DIGESTION
B
C
THIRD DIGESTION
LIVER
STOMACH
USABLE PARTS ACTED UPON BY DIGESTIVE FLUIDS
COLON
FOOD IN SMALL INTESTINE BECOMES CHYME BY MIXING WITH DIGESTIVE JUICES & INGESTED FLUIDS
UNUSABLE PARTS TO LARGE INTESTINE: EXCREMENT
D
FOURTH DIGESTION

ciples, it will be useful to present another arrangement of evaluating the heating and cooling properties of foods and spices, so that one may begin to make intelligent choices about the foods one consumes. It is hoped, *in shā' Allāh*, that one will see a remarkable improvement in health.

To facilitate the use of foods and herbs as medicines, all substances are classified according to their degree of heat or cold. There are four degrees of each, making a total of eight possible classifications for each food.

Thus a food or herb may be:

Hot in the First Degree		Cold in the First Degree
Hot in the Second Degree	or	Cold in the Second Degree
Hot in the Third Degree		Cold in the Third Degree
Hot in the Fourth Degree		Cold in the Fourth Degree

METABOLIC VALUES OF FOODS

Heating (Garmi) Foods

***Meat and Fish*:** lamb, liver, chicken, eggs, goat (male), fish (general)

***Dairy Products*:** sheep's milk, cream cheese, cream, clarified butter (ghee)

***Vegetables and Beans*:** beet, radish, onion, mustard greens, red lentils, white lentils, kidney beans, leek, eggplant, chick peas, red pepper, green pepper, carrot seed, squash

Fruits: banana, coconut, peach, plum, orange, lemon, mulberries, red raisins, green raisins, olive, ripe grapes, pumpkin, all dried fruits

***Seeds and Nuts*:** sesame, almond, pistachio, apricot kernels, walnut, pine nuts

***Grains*:** thin-grain rice, basmati rice

***Oils*:** sesame oil, corn oil, castor oil, mustard oil

***Beverages*:** black tea, coffee

***Herbs*:** cinnamon, cardamom, cloves, fenugreek, ginger, celery seed, anise seed, rue, saffron, garam masala (blend), curry powder (blend)

***Other*:** honey, rock candy, all sweet things, salt, all modern medicine

Cooling (Sardi) Foods

***Meat*:** rabbit, goat (female), beef

***Dairy Products*:** cow's milk, mother's milk, goat's milk, butter, buttermilk, dried cheeses, margarine

***Vegetables and Beans*:** lettuce, celery, sprouts (general), zucchini, spinach, cabbage, okra, cauliflower, broccoli, white potato, sweet potato, carrot, cucumber, soybeans, tomato, turnip, peas, beans (general)

Fruits: melons (general), pear, fig, pomegranate

***Seeds and Nuts*:** none

***Grains*:** brown rice, thick-grain rice

***Oils*:** sunflower oil, coconut oil

***Beverages*:** green teas

***Herbs*:** coriander (dry), dill, henna

Other: refined sugar, vinegar, bitter things, sour things

We learn from Avicenna that these degree have the following effects:

> First Degree: Affects metabolism, but not in any way discerned by physical sensation. Slightest action.
>
> Second Degree: Acts upon the body, causing metabolic change, but in the end is overwhelmed by the body. All nutrients belong to this category. Among the actions caused by second-degree substances are opening pores, initiating peristaltic action, causing perspiration, and stimulating digestion.
>
> Third Degree: Not acted upon by the body, but acts upon the body. All medicinal substances belong to this category. An example is senna pods, which overwhelm the eliminative powers and force rapid evacuation of the lower bowel.
>
> Fourth Degree: Causes cessation of metabolic function. Poisons are in this category. Some herbs are used as medicines from this category, but only in the most minute amounts and under the strict supervision of a physician.

By way of illustration, a second-degree hot substance would speed up metabolism, whereas a second-degree cold substance would slow it down. In the extreme fourth degree, a hot herb would cause an expansion of metabolism beyond the limits that support life, whereas a fourth-degree cold herb would slow down metabolism to the point of death.

An example of these principles in action is the common case of people eating curry that is too hot for them. Usually, they reach for a tall glass of water. However, this does not quench the burning, because water, in this system, is neutral. Instead, they should have on hand a small side dish of cucumbers and yogurt—two foods that are quite high in their cooling effect.

All elements of nature can be assigned a value according to this system of heating and cooling effects. And the diet can be adjusted according to all of the factors mentioned earlier: season, climate, altitude, prevalent illnesses, and so forth.

These dietary principles form the basis of all traditional societies and their eating habits. In the United States, those of Hispanic and African tribal origin have the vestiges of this system in their diet because both peoples were at one time part of Islamic culture.

The Sufi shaykh understands this system and frequently makes recommendations to correct a physical imbalance by introducing one or more foods. Each part of the body has its own characteristic degree of heat or cold—just as each of the four essences do—and so one can generally adjust the diet to raise or lower the metabolic balance.

For instance, a man may come before the shaykh complaining of painful joints—a condition called arthritis in Western terminology. The shaykh knows that the proper temperament of the interior nerves and joint fibers is somewhat cold and moist in a state of health. By observing the physical condition of the man, the shaykh will determine whether or not a cold or hot excess has created the imbalance, and he can prescribe an herb or food to correct the problem. This is similar to what a physician does, but the shaykh is also taking into account the effect of the *nafas*, or activator of the physiological actions.

When the breath is drawn in through the mouth and nostrils, it is destined to penetrate to the furthest reaches of each organ. True, the breath may undergo many changes before it reaches its goal, but it will always carry an intention to travel to the furthest reaches of all extremities. When a constriction occurs in the pathways of these breaths of life, disease conditions develop quickly. We could assign a value to the type of imbalance and peer inside the tissues to see that a particular bacteria thrived in the atmosphere of imbalance and grew to a larger than normal population. However, it is first of all necessary to unblock the constriction of the dispersal of the *nafas*—the life force itself. This accounts for the vast majority of miraculous cures of physical problems accomplished by the Sufis. The methods by which these blockages are unlocked will be taken up in a later chapter.

With all of the foregoing as a preface, we can now turn to study some of the specific knowledge of foods, as related by the master and guide of all Sufis, the Holy Prophet Muhammad (s.a.w.s.).

6

Foods of the Prophet (s.a.w.s.)

And the earth hath He appointed for
His creatures
Wherein are fruit and sheathed
palm trees,
Husked grain and scented herb.
Which is it of these favors of your Lord
that ye deny?

Qur'an 55:10–13

The Prophet Muhammad (s.a.w.s.) was once reported to have said, "There are two kinds of knowledge: knowledge of religion and knowledge of the body." The Prophet (s.a.w.s.) frequently commented upon the nature and value of various foods and spices. These comments were noted by his wives and companions (r.a.) and remain available to us today.

For the Sufi, the Prophet (s.a.w.s.) was the embodiment of one who lived as perfectly as possible, and as that includes his eating habits, his recommendations on diet form the basis of the Sufis' daily sustenance. At the beginning, the Sufi aspirant assumes a behavior known as *fanā' fī shaykh*—effacement in the shaykh. The period of following this course of behavior may be short or long. During this time, the *murīd* adopts as closely as possible the behavior of the shaykh in all respects. That is, the *murīd* dresses like the shaykh (or as the shaykh requests), eats the foods of the shaykh, takes up the practices advised by the shaykh. In short, the *murīd* dissolves himself in the image of the shaykh. The objective is for the *murīd* to discontinue his prior behavior and over time adapt himself to the character of the shaykh.

The point of this training, on one level, is to harmonize outward action with inward condition. This interaction is epitomized in three words: *īmān*, *islām*, and *iḥsān*. *Īmān* means to have true belief and absolute faith in God. When one possesses this requisite faith, it causes one to follow the commandments of God, called *sharī^cat*. The one who consciously follows these *sharīcat* laws is said to be living Islam.

When the way of life called *islām* is adhered to with finality, it causes the development of the interior stations of the soul, known as *iḥsān*, which means "blessing." On the Sufi path one cannot attain any of these conditions without the other; they are interdependent. As Sufi Abu Anees Barkat Ali once remarked: "Following the behavior of the Prophet (s.a.w.s.) is the *sunnah*, which is the root of Islam. Sufism is the fruit of the tree of Islam, or the fragrance of its fruit. If there is no root, how can there be any fruit?"

When this period of *fanā' fī shaykh* is ended, the *murīd* enters the next phase, called *fanā' fī murshid*, adopting the dress, foods, and general and specific behavior of the leader or *murshid* of the particular order to which the *murīd* belongs. Thus, the practices are extended, food is lessened and fasting increased, and the deeper meanings of the Qur'an are studied, revealed through the agency of the shaykhs of the order.

The next evolution is into that known as *fanā' fī rasūl*, in which, *in shā' Allāh*, the *murīd* is effaced in the image of the *rasūl Allah*, the Holy Prophet Muhammad (s.a.w.s.). Ultimately, following this stage, if successful, the *murīd* attains the state known as *fanā' fī Llāh*, or total annihilation in the Almighty.

Because the Sufi path is a gradual and reasonable one, fully in accord with human nature in every regard, the *murīd* at the outset concentrates upon adopting the correct manner of eating, sleeping, walking, sitting, praying, and similar behaviors. At all times, the shaykh holds sway over the *murīd*, to offer helpful suggestions and guidance, and to correct kindly any actions that the *murīd* may do incorrectly.

In the earlier stages of Sufism, the struggle is mainly to subdue the gross physical appetites of the *nafs*, and therefore, the following statements and suggestions of the Prophet Muhammad (s.a.w.s.), which also include some of the knowledge associated with the physicians of Islam, become vital for every aspirant to learn, understand, and apply.

Before presenting a selection of the Hadith specifically relating to health, it is necessary to reflect for a moment on the nature of some of these recommendations. To some people, the advice which follows may seem quaint, old-fashioned, or simply bizarre. Some may feel that a particular statement has not been or cannot be confirmed by scientific knowledge. However, all of the statements and actions of the Prophet (s.a.w.s.) are woven upon the nucleus of divine inspiration, and so do not admit of any error, inaccuracy, or amendment. A few illustrations will make this clear.

There is a Hadith that says that if a fly falls into a liquid while one is preparing to drink it, the person should first dip the fly completely under the surface of the water and submerge the fly totally before removing it. This advice seems very strange, if not dangerous.

Medically it is known that a fly carries some pathogens on some parts of its body (this was mentioned by the Prophet Muhammad [s.a.w.s.] 1,400 years ago, when there was practically no formal medical knowledge). But Allah has said that He created no disease without also creating its remedy, except death (meaning the decline of old age). Therefore, in modern times penicillin has been discovered, which is used to counteract harmful organisms such as staphylococci. However, Dr. Muhammad M. el-Samahy, director of the Department of Hadith at al-Azhar University at Cairo, Egypt, has written an article revealing the astute medical genius of this apparently mysterious advice.

Dr. el-Samahy relates that microbiologists have discovered that there are longitudinal cells living as parasites inside the stomach of the fly. These yeast cells, as part of their own reproductive cycle, protrude through the respiratory tubules of the fly. When the fly is dipped completely into a liquid, the resulting change in the osmotic pressure causes the cells to burst. The contents of those cells is an antidote for pathogens which the fly carries on its body. Thus, the latest research in microbiology confirms what has been known from Prophetic knowledge for 1,400 years.

Another example concerns the advice to take a small amount of salt before beginning a meal. This in particular seems to be contradicted by modern medical wisdom, which stresses the harmful effects of excess salt consumption. However, a knowledge of the metabolism of the body illustrates the wisdom of this suggestion as well.

Salt is composed of two chemicals: sodium and chloride. The chlorides present in salt constitute the only readily available source of chlorides with which the body can manufacture hydrochloric acid, vital for proper digestion in the stomach. Thus, taking in a small amount of salt prior to the meal allows any deficiency of hydrochloric acid to be made up just before introducing new food.

It should be added that the harmful effects of excess salt are primarily associated with raised levels of sodium, not chlorides. In fact, persons who eliminate salt entirely from their diet may be subject to further disease caused by lack of proper levels of hydrochloric acid.

These two examples prove that there is indeed intelligent medical reasoning for following the recommendations of these Hadith. It is true that not all of these Hadith have been submitted to scientific confirmation. It must be pointed out, however, that even if scientific experiments were done to confirm each and every statement, the fact that science did not, or could not, confirm its value would not negate the truth of the statement.

For scientific knowledge is constantly changing, and too often experiments have been found to be done incorrectly, and even intentionally falsified. For the Sufi, it is sufficient that God has mentioned, or inspired His Prophet (s.a.w.s.) to advise, a practice. Human knowledge or experience can never contradict or amend the divine knowledge and commandments.

Once these words of advice are integrated into dietary habits, one will discover that every action is perfectly in accord with human nature, and immènse health benefits will accrue to anyone applying them with sincerity.

Not only can various recipes be gleaned from the commentaries that follow, but also individual foods and herbs are often prescribed as medicines.

It is impossible to state with finality which food or herb would be given in a particular case, because the person must be present before the healer or physician, in order for him to make a correct diagnosis of the imbalance. Nonetheless, the foods discussed in the following sections should be preferred over others, and the suggestions for combining them adhered to.*

It must be remembered that it is not simply the eating of one or more foods that marks the Sufi's behavior. There are many other aspects of behavior that bear upon health—fasting, prayer, giving of alms, and other practices—and these other factors may have a greater total impact on health than any foods.

SAYINGS OF THE PROPHET (s.a.w.s.)

Before proceeding to the listing of foods, it is worthwhile to provide the statements of the Prophet (s.a.w.s.) relating to manners, hygiene, prevention, and similar topics, bearing on health.

Said the Prophet of Allah (s.a.w.s.):

Allah did not create any illness without also creating the remedy, except death [old age]. Allah said that he who lives according to the Qur'an will have a long life.

The origin of every disease is cold. So eat when you desire and refrain when you desire.

The stomach is the home of disease and abstinence the head of every remedy. So make this your custom.

In the sight of Allah, the best food is a food shared by many.

To eat the morning meal alone is to eat with satan; to eat with one other person is to eat with a tyrant; to eat with two other persons is to eat with the prophets (peace be upon them all).

*In my judgment, the cuisine of Afghanistan provides the best recipes for applying all of these foods in proper proportion, and in that country, at least, the foods are eaten in light of availability by season. Unfortunately, there are few easily obtainable books on Afghan cooking. It is also a fact that the men and women of Afghanistan are probably among the most vigorous and hearty and pious on earth.

Allow your food to cool before eating, for in hot food there is no blessing.

When you eat, take your shoes off, for then indeed your feet have more rest. This is an excellent advice.

There is blessing in the middle of a dish. So commence from the side and not from the middle.*

There is blessing in three things: in the early morning meal, in bread and in soup.

Brush your teeth with a *miswāk* [a wooden toothpick usually made from a twig of the pelu tree] after a meal and rinse out your mouth. For these two practices are a safeguard for the eyeteeth and the wisdom teeth.

Use *miswāk*, for this practice comes from cleanliness, and cleanliness comes from faith, and faith takes its practitioner to heaven.

The dish pleads for mercy for the one who takes up the last morsel [i.e., do not be wasteful].

Eat together and then disperse, for a blessing resides in groups.

Less food, less sin.

To horde in these things is unlawful: wheat, barley, raisins, millet, fats, honey, cheese, walnuts, and olives.

Let no one drink while standing up, except one who is suffering from sciatica.

Eat your meal at dawn, for there is blessing in a meal at dawn.

When I was taken up into Heaven, I did not pass one angel who did not say to me: "O Muhammad, tell your people to make use of scarification [allowing out a small amount of blood from an incision]. The best treatment that you have is scarification, coriander, and costus [an East Indian herb].

Whoever is sick for seven days, thereby he expiates before Allah the sins of seventy years.

There is no pain like pain in the eye, and no worry like the worry of a debt.

When the Prophet (s.a.w.s.) came before a sick person, he used to say: "Get rid of evil delusions. Strength is with Allah the Almighty. Cure and be cured. There is no healing but Yours."

*The implication here is that one should exhibit a selfless reserve and allow another to obtain the blessing, not hog it for oneself.

LIST OF FOODS

Aniseed (*anīsūn*)—Among its many properties, the seed of anise soothes internal pains, increases menstrual flow, promotes secretion of milk and semen, and dissolves intestinal gas. It may be applied in tea form to the eyes to strengthen eyesight. In nature, snakes coming out of winter hibernation seek out the anise plant and rub their eyes against it, because their vision becomes weak over winter.

Apple (*tuffāḥ*)—Sour apples are more cooling than sweet ones. It is claimed that apples strengthen the heart.

Asparagus (*hiyawn*)—Hot and moist, asparagus opens obstructions of the kidneys and eases childbirth. It is said that asparagus will kill dogs that eat it.

Banana (*mawz*)—Hot in the first degree, banana has little use as a food, except for people with a very cold intemperament, who should eat it with honey.

Barley (*shaᶜīr*)—Barley ranks below only wheat as a desirable food. It is the first recommendation for hot intemperament diseases. Barley is soaked in water, which is drunk for coughs and sore throats. The Prophet (s.a.w.s.) always gave a soup made from barley to anyone suffering from the pain of fever.

Basil, Sweet (*rayḥān*)—Smelling basil strengthens the heart. Sleep is promoted by rubbing the head with basil and water.

Bread (*khubz*)—The best bread is made of the finest whole grain flours and is baked in a circular stone oven. Bread should be allowed to cool somewhat before being eaten, or it will make one excessively thirsty. Stale bread clogs the bowels. Bread containing substantial bran is digested quickly, but is very nourishing. The softer the bread, the easier the digestion and the greater the nourishment. Bread crumbs produce gas. Breads made from barley and pea flours are slow to be digested and must have salt added to them. Said the Prophet (s.a.w.s.): "Do not cut bread with a knife, but give it due honor by breaking it with the hands, for Allah has honored it."

Butter (*zubdah*)—Butter is mildly hot and moist. Useful to alleviate constipation, butter is also mixed with honey and dates to make a food that removes the food cravings of pregnant women.

Cauliflower (*qunnabīṭ*)—This vegetable is hard to digest, and it is said to harm the vision.

Chamomile (*bābūnaj*)—Hot in the first degree, chamomile is mild. Its main use is to promote urination and menstrual flow.

Carrot (*jazar*)—Sexual urges arise from eating carrot, which is hot in the second degree. It also is used to increase menstrual flow and urination.

Coconut *(nārjīl darja'i)*—The best type is very white, which is hot and moist. The nature of coconut is that it increases sexual powers and relieves pain in the back.

Coffee Bean (*qahwah*)—Coffee is a corrective for dysentery, relieves thirst, and is said to produce wisdom. It should be used sparingly.

Coriander Seed (*ḥabb al-suda*)—The most respected books of traditions state that the Prophet (s.a.w.s.) said, "Make yours the seeds of coriander, for it is a cure of all diseases except swelling [cancer], and that is a fatal disease." It is also reported that Allah informed the Prophet, "She has been given everything." And then Allah revealed that "she" is coriander. Coriander alleviates flatulence and resolves fevers. It is effective in the treatment of leukoderma, and it opens the subtlest networks of the veins. Excess moisture in the body is dried up by coriander, and it increases milk flow, urine, and menses. It is particularly useful when a person has a cold. The oil of coriander is a treatment for baldness and scalp problems, and prevents gray hair. The smoke of the burning seeds is an insect repellent.

Chicken (*dajaj*)—Light on the stomach and easy to digest, chicken is the best of fowl meats. It corrects and balances all the essences, is a food that is good for the brain, and improves the complexion. However, overconsumption of chicken leads to gout. The best chicken is a hen that has never laid an egg.

Cinnamon (*darchini*)—Cinnamon is hot in the third degree. Its volatile oil is a great medicine for indigestion. It forms an ingredient in spice blends used as the basis of cooking in almost three-fourths of the world.

Citron (*utrujj*)—The Prophet (s.a.w.s.) is reported to have said, "The citron is like a true believer: good to taste and good to smell." Citron strengthens the heart, dispels sadness, removes freckles, satisfies hunger, and slows the flow of bile. The wife of the Prophet (s.a.w.s.) used to treat blind persons with citron dipped in honey. Citron is best taken about ten minutes after the conclusion of meals.

Cucumber (*qiṭṭā'*)—Ripe cucumbers dispel heat and are diuretic. Eating dates with green cucumber is said to cause weight gain.

Cumin (*kammūn*)—Cumin is very hot. It is reported to be the only spice or herb that travels through the stomach unaffected by digestion, until it reaches the liver. Cumin soaked in water, which is then drunk, is excellent for colic.

Dates, Dried (*tamr*)—The Prophet (s.a.w.s.) is reported to have said, "A house without dates has no food." Prophet Muhammad (s.a.w.s.) used to plant date trees himself. Dates should be eaten with almonds to annul any adverse effects. Fresh dates were the food eaten by Mary (r.a.), at the time of her delivery of the infant Jesus (a.s.). Said the Prophet (s.a.w.s.), "He who finds a date, let him break his fast on that. If he finds no date, let him break it on water. For verily that is purity."

Eggplant (*bādhinjān*)—The dark variety of eggplant causes production of bile. Small amounts of it help piles. Eggplant's tendency to produce bile is corrected by eating it with meat dishes.

Eggs (*bayḍah*)—The best eggs are those of chickens, eaten soft, not hard-boiled. Egg white relieves pain of sunburn, aids healing of burns, and prevents scarring. Eggs are aphrodisiac.

Endive (*hindibā'*)—The effects of endive change according to the season. Endive at the earliest time is best, and at the end of the growing season, virtually useless. The Hadith states: "Eat endives and do not belch, for verily there is not one day that drops of the water of Paradise do not fall upon them [endives]."

Fenugreek (*ḥulbah*)—It is reported the Prophet (s.a.w.s.) once said: "If my people knew what there is in fenugreek, they would have bought and paid its weight in gold." Fenugreek is hot and dry. As a tea it aids menstrual flow and is useful in colic and as a cleansing enema. Fenugreek strengthens the heart.

Fig (*tin*)—Fresh figs are preferred to dried. Although quite nourishing, they are very hot. The Prophet (s.a.w.s.) is reported to have said, "If you say that any fruit has come from Paradise, then you must mention the fig, for indeed it is the fruit of Paradise. So eat of it, for it is a cure for piles and helps gout."

Fish (*samak*)—Fresh-water fish are best, and those which feed on plant life, not mud and effluvia. Uncooked fish is hard to digest and produces imbalance of phlegm.

Garlic (*thawm*)—Garlic is hot in the third degree. It is used to dispel gas, promote menses, and expel afterbirth. It is excellent to correct cold intemperament, for dissolving phlegm, and the oil is used to treat insect bites. The eating of raw garlic and then visiting the mosque has been forbidden by the Prophet Muhammad (s.a.w.s.).

Ghee (clarified butter) (*samn*)—Ghee is the most fatty of all condiments. It is to be considered a medicinal additive to foods. Mixed with honey, ghee is said to be an antidote to poisons.

Ginger (*zanjabīl*)—Ginger is mentioned in the Holy Qur'an (76:17). It is hot in the third degree, and is best for softening phlegm. It also aids digestion and strengthens sexual activity.

Henna (*ḥinnā'*)—One Hadith reports that nothing is dearer to Allah than henna. The Holy Prophet (s.a.w.s.) recommended it for many conditions: bruises, pain in the legs, infection of nails, burns, and to beautify the hair. Henna is noted for its great heat and its ability to excite the passions of love. The perfume made from henna flowers is considered to be one of the finest in the world. The dyeing of hands, nails, and feet is a common practice in the East, especially for weddings and feasts.

Honey (*ᶜasal*)—Allah has said: "There comes forth, from within [the bee], a beverage of many colors in which there is a healing for you." Mixed with hot water, and taken in several small doses, honey is considered the best remedy for diarrhea.

The Prophet (s.a.w.s.) once said, "By Him in whose hand is my soul, eat honey. For there is no house in which honey is kept for which the angels will not ask for mercy. If a person eats honey, a thousand remedies enter his stomach and a million diseases will come out. If a man dies and honey is found within him, fire will not touch his body [i.e., he will be immune from the burning of hell]." The Prophet (s.a.w.s.) himself used to drink a glass of honey and water each morning on an empty stomach.

Honey is considered the food of foods, the drink of drinks, and the drug of drugs. It is used for creating appetite, strengthening the stomach, and eliminating phlegm; as a meat preservative, hair conditioner, eye salve, and mouthwash. The best honey is that produced in the spring; the second best is that of summer, and the least quality is produced in winter.

Lentils (*ʿadas*)—All lentils produce dryness. Small amounts should be eaten, as a side dish, for in quantity they are generally bad for the stomach. Hadith say that the eating of lentils produces a sympathetic heart, tears in the eyes, and removes pride.

Lettuce (*khass*)—Although cold, lettuce is considered the best nourishment of all vegetables. It softens a hard constitution and helps those who suffer delirium. It contradicts the sexual energy and dries up semen. Excess consumption of lettuce weakens the eyesight.

Marjoram, Sweet (*marzanjūsh*)—The Prophet (s.a.w.s.) is reported to have said that sweet marjoram is most excellent for anyone who has lost the sense of smell.

Meat (*laḥm*)—Allah has said in the Qur'an (52:22): "And we will aid them with fruit and meat, such as they desire." The Prophet (s.a.w.s.) reportedly said that one who does not eat meat for forty consecutive days will waste away, whereas to eat meat for forty consecutive days will harden the heart. In other words, one should moderate the intake of meat.

The most desirable of all meats is mutton, which is hot and moist in temperament. The best mutton is that of a male yearling; the best cut is a shoulder roast. Mutton should be cooked in some liquid, or it tends to dry out.

Beef fat mixed with pepper and cinnamon acts as a tonic medicine. The meat of pigs is forbidden to eat. The consumption of horse flesh as a food is disputed. Avicenna said the flesh of camels, horses, and asses are the worst of all meats. Also prohibited for human consumption are beasts of prey, animals that possess canine teeth, and birds with hooked talons.

Said the Prophet (s.a.w.s.): "Do not cut up meat with a knife upon the dish, for that is the way of non-Muslims. But grasp it in your fingers and so it will taste better." And, he said: "One sheep is a blessing; two sheep are two blessings; three sheep are wealth."

Melon (*baṭṭīkh*)—Said the Prophet (s.a.w.s.): "Whenever you eat fruit, eat melon, because it is the fruit of Paradise and contains a thousand blessings and a thousand mercies. The eating of it cures every disease." Generally, the sweeter a melon, the greater its heat. Green varieties tend to be cold; the yellow, hot. The Prophet took melons with fresh dates. Melon purifies the bladder and the stomach, and improves the spinal fluid and eyesight. Melons should not be eaten first in a meal. Said the Prophet (s.a.w.s.): "None of your women who are pregnant and eat of watermelon will fail to produce offspring who are good in countenance and good in character."

Milk (*laban*)—Allah has mentioned milk to us, saying, "Rivers of milk the taste whereof does not change" (Qur'an 47:15). And again He said, "Pure milk, easy and agreeable to swallow for those who drink" (Qur'an 16:66). The Prophet Muhammad (s.a.w.s.) is said to have remarked that milk is irreplaceable and that he himself loved milk.

Milk is composed of fat and water and milk solids (cheese). Together, these components are well suited to the constitution of humans. However, we should not take the milk of animals whose pregnancy lasts longer than that of humans. The milk of cows is best, for they feed off grasses.

Said the Prophet (s.a.w.s.): "Drink milk, for it wipes away heat from the heart as the finger wipes away sweat from the brow. Furthermore, it strengthens the back, increases the brain, augments the intelligence, renews vision, and drives away forgetfulness."

A milk diet is the best treatment there is for dropsy; however, anyone with fever must avoid milk.

Mint (*na^{c}na^c*)—The most subtle and refined of pot herbs, mint is heating and drying. Mint strengthens the stomach, cures hiccups, and encourages sexual activity. Placed in milk, mint will prevent it from turning to cheese.

Myrtle (*ās*)—Cold in the second degree, myrtle is most used to stem diarrhea. Smelling the oil will cure headache caused by overheating. Myrtle tea with quince added is used for coughs.

Narcissus (*narjis*)—One Hadith says, "Smell a narcissus, even if only once a day or once a week or once a month or once a year or once a lifetime. For verily in the heart of man there is the seed of insanity, leprosy, and leukoderma. And the scent of narcissus drives them away."

Olives and Olive Oil (*zayt* and *zaytūn*)—The older olive oil is, the hotter it becomes. Olive oil is an excellent treatment for the skin and hair, and it delays old age.

Allah has said of the olive tree: "And a tree that grows out of Mount Sinai which produces oil and a condiment for those who eat. For olive oil is the supreme seasoning." Allah has also called it the Blessed Tree (Qur'an 24:35).

Green olives are the most nourishing, and counteract autointoxication. Black olives cause the spleen to overproduce bile and are hard on the stomach. Olive leaves can be chewed as treatment for inflammation of the stomach, skin ulcerations, and eruptions of herpes and hives.

Onion (*baṣal*)—Quite hot, the onion is a good corrective for all excess wetness. Onion improves the flavor of foods and eliminates phlegm. Raw onions cause forgetfulness. An excess of cooked onions causes headache and forgetfulness.

Parsley (*karafs*)—A Hadith states that eating parsley just before sleep will cause one to awaken with sweet breath and will eliminate or prevent toothache. Parsley stimulates sexual activity.

Peach (*khu'kh*)—Peaches generate cold, relax the stomach, and soften the bowels. A good laxative, peaches should be eaten before, rather than after, a meal.

Pistachio (*fustaq*)—It is said that to eat the heart of a pistachio nut with egg yolk will make the heart grow strong. The reddish skin stems diarrhea and vomiting.

Pomegranate (*rummān*)—Sweet pomegranates are preferred over the sour. The juice stems coughs. All kinds of pomegranates settle palpitations of the heart. Hazrat ᶜAlī (r.a.) said that the light of Allah is in the heart of whoever eats pomegranates. It is also reported that one who eats three pomegranates in the course of a year will be inoculated against ophthalmia for that year.

Said the Prophet (s.a.w.s.): Pomegranate "cleanses you of Satan and from evil aspirations for forty days."

Quince (*safarjal*)—It is said that to eat quince on an empty stomach is good for the soul. Cold and dry, quince is astringent to the stomach, and it checks excessive menstrual flow. A few seeds placed in water will, after a few minutes, form a mucilage which is an excellent remedy for cough and sore throat, especially in the young. Quince is also excellent for pregnant women, gladdening their hearts. The Holy Prophet (s.a.w.s.) said: "Eat quince, for it sweetens the heart. For Allah has sent no prophet as His messenger without feeding him on the quince of Paradise. For quince increases the strength up to that of forty men."

Rhubarb (*rāwand*)—Rhubarb is hot and dry, and best when picked fresh. It opens blockages of the liver and resolves chronic fever.

Rice (*aruzz*)—Next to wheat, rice is the most nourishing of whole grain foods. It is said eating rice increases pleasant dreams and the production of semen. Eating rice cooked in fat from sheep's liver is better and more effective than a major purging.

Saffron (*za^{c}farān*)—Hot and dry, saffron is excellent for the blood and strengthening to the soul. It eases pains in the joints, but can cause great increase in the sex drive of young men.

Salt (*milḥ*)—Hot and dry in the third degree, salt, when taken moderately, is beautifying to the skin, giving it a soft glow. Salt causes vomiting when purging, and stimulates the appetite. Excessive use causes the skin to itch.

The Prophet (s.a.w.s.) recommended beginning and ending each meal with a pinch of salt. He said: "From the one who begins a meal with salt, Allah wards off three hundred and thirty kinds of diseases, the least of which are lunacy, leprosy, bowel troubles, and toothache. The rest is prescribed in the supreme knowledge of Allah."

Senna (*sanā*)—The best species of henna is that from the blessed city of Medina, where it grows plentifully. The chief property of senna is that it strengthens the heart without harshness. Its nobility has caused it to be referred to by the *ḥakīms* as the Glory of Drugs. Its uses are many—in purgative infusions, decoctions, pills, enemas, and powders. Senna causes the bile to flow, and reaches to the very depths of the joints to balance the essences therein. The most effective use is as a tea, which can be made even more efficacious by adding violet blossoms and crushed red raisins. The Prophet (s.a.w.s.) recommended senna most highly, making a statement similar to the one about coriander: that it cures every disease except death itself.

Spinach (*asfānākh*)—Spinach is cold and moist, causing irritation to the chest and throat. Still, it softens the bowels.

Sugar (*sukkar*)—Sugar is cold and moist. It is most often used in combination with other medicinal herbs, which carry the effects to the furthest point of an organ. Eating too much sugar creates disease of moisture.

Thyme (*ṣa^{c}tar*)—In the time of the Prophet (s.a.w.s.), it was customary to fumigate houses by burning frankincense and thyme. Thyme is cold and dry in the third degree. An excellent digestive aid to heavy foods, thyme beautifies the complexion, annuls intestinal gas, and benefits coldness of the stomach and liver. When drunk as an infusion, it is said to kill tapeworms.

Vermicelli (*iṭriyyah*)—This food is hot and excessively moist, thus hard to digest. For those with very strong constitution, it provides excellent nourishment.

Vinegar (*khall*)—The Prophet Muhammad (s.a.w.s.) was reported to have once remarked that vinegar was the seasoning of all the prophets who came before him. Vinegar is both cold and hot, nearly balanced between the two. Mixed with rose water, it is an excellent remedy for toothache and headache. Vinegar dissolves phlegm. Another Hadith states that a house containing vinegar will never suffer from poverty.

Walnut (*jawz*)—Walnut is the hottest of nuts. Although hard to digest, when eaten with raisins it is the best remedy for winter cough. Avicenna said that walnuts cure the effects of poisons.

Water (*mā'*)—The Prophet (s.a.w.s.) reportedly said: "The best drink in this world and the next is water." Water is moist and, because of this, slightly cooling. It extinguishes thirst and preserves the innate moisture of the body. It assists digestion of foods and absorption of nutrients. Said the Prophet (s.a.w.s.): "When you have a thirst, drink [water] by sips and do not gulp it down. . . . Gulping water produces sickness of the liver."

Wheat (*ḥinṭah*)—Wheat is somewhat hot, and balanced between dryness and moisture. The eating of raw wheat produces intestinal worms and gas. Wheat flour should be ground during the daytime.

So praise be upon this unlettered Prophet who produced for us this marvelous knowledge which makes us see and understand and dazzles the wisest minds. Herein are proofs of God's kindness and benevolence upon His creatures, for He is the most kind and all-loving. May we serve Him with true vision.

Al-ḥamdu li-Lāhi Rabb il-ᶜĀlamīn!
So all praise be to Allah,
Lord of the Worlds! ***Āmīn!***

7

Herbal Formulas for Common Ailments

O mankind! There hath come to you
a direction from your Lord
And a healing for the diseases in
your hearts—
And for those who believe,
a Guidance, and a Mercy.

Qur'an 10:57

It is the custom of the shaykhs to first of all resort to some form of dietary advice to effect the cure of simple imbalances. This dietary reform may include adjusting the use of various herbs and spices in cooking.

The herbal formulas given in this chapter make use of the foods, herbs, and spices presented in the foregoing chapters. They are usually easy to obtain and require very little effort to prepare. These remedies are formulated according to the qualities of heat and coldness (*garmi* and *sardi*) of each substance and work primarily by rebalancing the temperament of one or more of the four essences of the body. Despite their simplicity, these herbal formulas are quite effective.

Preparation of Remedies

1. Formulas should be prepared according to instructions.
2. When a formula calls for *powdered* herbs, they should be ground to a fine powder and sieved through a muslin cloth or a sieve of 100 mesh (unless formula says a coarse powder may be used).
3. When herbs are to be made into a decoction (boiled in water), as soon as the water starts to boil, the vessel should be removed from the fire and allowed to sit for five minutes; then the liquid should be strained and drunk warm.
4. When a formula calls for a liquid to be *reduced to half*, the vessel should be kept on a medium fire until about half the water has evaporated by boiling.

DOSAGE

Adults (above age fifteen) should be given a full dose. Children may be given the following amounts according to age:

Up to one year	Consult physician
1–2 years	1/6 of adult dose
3–4 years	1/4 of adult dose
5–6 years	1/3 of adult dose
7–9 years	1/2 of adult dose
10–15 years	3/4 of adult dose

WEIGHTS AND MEASURES

1 tablespoon	=	3 teaspoons
1 cup	=	8 fluid ounces
1 pint	=	2 cups
1 quart	=	2 pints
1 gallon	=	4 quarts
1 centiliter	=	0.34 fluid ounce
1 deciliter	=	3.38 fluid ounces
1 liter	=	1.06 quarts
1 decaliter	=	2.64 gallons
Less than a teaspoon	=	a few grains
1 teaspoon	=	1 dram
1 tablespoon	=	4 drams
1 teacup	=	7 ounces

5. Sugar, if it is to be added to a formula, should be a fine powder of pure, raw, unrefined sugar, such as that from Mexico. If unavailable, use honey in its place.
6. In some cases, the instructions say to soak an herb overnight. If this cannot be done, the herbs may be soaked for three to four hours, and then simmered five to six hours before using. This method would also be used in winter.
7. When instructed to make a "water" (e.g., ginger water, lime water), soak one to two ounces of the herb or other substance in one pint of pure water for four to six hours. Strain before using.

8. Formulas that are to be preserved and used for more than one day may also be prepared in reduced or lesser quantities than called for. The ratios of each ingredient must be carefully adjusted in such cases.
9. When *equal parts* of herbs are to be used, each herb should be equal by weight or volume. The quantity to be taken should be decided in light of the dose recommended and the number of days for which the formula is to be prepared at one time.

Storage

1. Decoctions are to be prepared fresh for single doses. Doses should not be made in the morning for evening consumption, or vice versa.
2. Do not expose remedies to direct sunlight, unless that is part of the method of preparation.
3. Containers should be cleaned and dried completely in the sun before formulas are stored in them. Never store herbal formulas in open containers.
4. If a formula is to be kept for more than one day, store it in a well-sealed glass bottle.
5. *Label all formulas,* especially those that are for external use only. Keep all herbal formulas out of the reach of children. Safety caps are advised for all bottles.

Administration

1. Remedies are usually taken twice daily, unless otherwise stated. Morning dose should be taken after a light breakfast, and evening dose between 4:00 and 6:00 P.M.
2. Remedies to be taken in the morning should be taken on an empty stomach, immediately after rising and performing toilet and cleansing.
3. Herb preparations to be taken after meals should be consumed five to fifteen minutes after eating a main meal.
4. Formulas to be taken at bedtime should be taken two hours after the evening meal.
5. The quantity indicated to be "taken as such" is meant to be a single dose.
6. Vehicles such as milk, water, soda water, and tea have been mentioned for some formulas. In such cases, the vehicle usually is one cup, unless stated otherwise.
7. Where no vehicles are mentioned, the remedy should be taken with water (in winter, with lukewarm water).

Caution: Some of the formulas use rose petals. Almost all commercially grown roses are treated with toxic chemicals. Use *only* organically grown roses in these formulas. If in doubt, use another formula.

THE FORMULARY

ANEMIA

Paleness of whole body, eyes, and fingernail beds. Swelling of face and feet, especially in the morning. General weakness, giddiness, loss of appetite, and sometimes diarrhea.

Instructions: Light diet, with fresh fruits and foods such as chicken soup, liver extract, beets, carrots, spinach, and fenugreek, is advised. Avoid fatty foods.

FORMULA 1

6 teaspoons fennel seeds, crushed
6 teaspoons red rose petals

Preparation: Boil in 1 1/2 cups water and strain.
Dosage: Twice daily.

FORMULA 2

4 teaspoons ground Indian cinnamon
8 teaspoons honey
8 cups pomegranate juice

Preparation: Dissolve cinnamon and honey in pomegranate juice.
Dosage: 2 teaspoons in 1/2 cup of water, as needed.

FORMULA 3

1 teaspoon purslane
1 teaspoon sweet basil
1 teaspoon gum arabic
9 teaspoons olive oil
1 cup rose water

Preparation: Fry first three ingredients in olive oil for ten minutes. Remove and soak in rose water for one hour.
Dosage: 1 teaspoon several times per day.

ANGINA PECTORIS

Pain in the chest muscles in the area of the heart, due to cold (*sardi*) imbalance.

Instructions: Avoid exposure to cold air.

FORMULA 1

1 teaspoon fenugreek
2 teaspoons honey

Preparation: Boil fenugreek in 1 1/2 cups of water, strain, and add honey.
Dosage: Twice daily.

FORMULA 2

1 teaspoon rose oil
4 teaspoons sweet almond oil

Preparation: Thoroughly mix two oils together.
Dosage: Rub on chest, morning and evening.

ARTHRITIS

There is pain and/or stiffness, without swelling, in one or more joints. Sometimes fever.

Instructions: Avoid sour and spicy (*garmi*) foods. Take walks in the morning, but avoid exposure to very cold air.

External Treatment: Rub with oil of amber and frankincense.

FORMULA 1

1 teaspoon powdered valerian root
1 teaspoon chamomile
1/2 teaspoon hops
1 teaspoon hay saffron

Preparation: Mix first three ingredients in 3 cups water and bring to boil. Remove from heat at first sign of boiling. Add saffron and steep for twenty minutes. Strain.
Dosage: 1/2 to 1 cup before bedtime.

FORMULA 2

6 teaspoons ginger
6 teaspoons caraway seeds
3 teaspoons black pepper

Preparation: Combine into a fine powder and preserve.
Dosage: 1/2 teaspoon with water, twice daily.

ASTHMA

Asthma occurs in spasmodic attacks of difficult breathing. When experiencing the asthma attack, the person should sit forward with the head resting on the hands and elbows on the knees. The face turns pale, and there is a wheezing sound in the breath. After extended coughing, the person usually emits a small amount of phlegm.

Instructions: Avoid exposure to cold air. Avoid cold (*sardi*) and sour foods.

External Treatment: Rub chest with oil of sweet almond.

FORMULA 1

1 teaspoon ground ginger

Preparation: Pour 1 1/2 cups hot water over the ginger.
Dosage: One teaspoon, lukewarm, at bedtime.

FORMULA 2

1/2 teaspoon skunk cabbage
1/2 teaspoon horehound
1/2 teaspoon cayenne pepper
1/2 teaspoon bayberry bark
1/2 teaspoon powdered valerian root
3 ounces molasses

Preparation: Grind all herbs fine and mix with molasses.
Dosage: 1 teaspoon in cup of hot tea, as needed.

BEDWETTING

FORMULA 1

1 teaspoon pomegranate flowers
1 teaspoon ground sesame seeds
1 teaspoon gum acacia
1 teaspoon crushed coriander seeds
Dark brown sugar (*gur*), as needed

Preparation: Fry coriander seeds in a cast-iron skillet until they are lightly burned. Mix in other ingredients, except brown sugar, and make a fine powder. Add brown sugar to equal the amount of powdered herbs.
Dosage: 1 teaspoon at bedtime.

FORMULA 2

3 teaspoons ground dried water chestnut
3 teaspoons raw sugar

Preparation: Make a fine powder of dried water chestnut and mix with sugar.
Dosage: 1 teaspoon, twice daily.

FORMULA 3

1 teaspoon cumin
1 teaspoon ground cloves
1 teaspoon mastic herb
3 ounces honey

Preparation: Grind and mix the first three ingredients, add honey, and mix well.
Dosage: 1 teaspoon, morning and evening.

BRONCHITIS IN CHILDREN

Breathing is rapid, and there is a hollow sound beneath the ribs while breathing. Cough, pain, and high fever are often present. Face becomes red and nostrils dilate while breathing. Child becomes restless.
Instructions: Avoid exposure to cold air. Take liquid diet.

FORMULA 1

2 teaspoons cut licorice root
2 teaspoons linseed
12 teaspoons honey

Preparation: Boil the first two herbs in 1 1/2 cups water for ten minutes. Strain and sweeten with honey.
Dosage: Two to three times per day.

FORMULA 2

1/8 teaspoon aloe

Preparation: Dissolve in mother's milk or cow's milk.
Dosage: (1) Administer to child as such. (2) Dissolve aloe in lukewarm water and apply on the chest.

FORMULA 3

1 teaspoon oil of garlic
3 teaspoons honey

Preparation: Mix ingredients together.
Dosage: Allow child to lick up a small amount with tongue, three times per day.

BURNS AND SCALDS

FORMULA 1

Pomegranate flowers, as needed.

Preparation and Administration: Grind with water to make a paste and apply on affected part.

FORMULA 2

4 teaspoons lime water
4 teaspoons coconut oil

Preparation and Administration: Combine and rub until mixture turns white; then apply on affected parts.

FORMULA 3

1 egg white

Preparation and Administration: Apply to affected parts. Especially effective if blister has appeared.

COLIC

Acute pain in abdomen and constipation. Abdomen is distended. Flatulence and gurgling sound are present.
External Treatment: Massage body with rose oil or sweet almond oil.
Recommended Foods: Green pea soup, chicken soup.

FORMULA 1

2 teaspoons wild basil

Preparation and Administration: Grind with water to make a paste, and apply to abdomen.

FORMULA 2

1 drop oil of peppermint
or
1 teaspoon peppermint leaves

Preparation: Mix peppermint oil in 6–8 ounces water; or boil leaves in 1 cup water for three minutes.
Dosage: Drink glassful twice daily.

FORMULA 3

6 ounces rose water, honey water, or fennel water

Dosage: Drink once per day.

COMMON COLD

Attacks of sneezing, watery discharge from nose, headache, cough, malaise, sometimes mild fever.

FORMULA 1

1 teaspoon violet flowers

Preparation: Boil for three minutes in 1 cup of water and strain.
Dosage: Twice daily on empty stomach.

FORMULA 2

1 teaspoon wheat husk
5 black peppercorns
1/6 teaspoon salt

Preparation: Boil ingredients in 1 cup water for three minutes, and strain.
Dosage: Twice daily.

FORMULA 3

1/2 teaspoon cinnamon bark, broken into bits

Preparation: Boil in 1 1/2 cups water for ten minutes, strain, and sweeten with honey.
Dosage: Twice daily.

CONSTIPATION

Instructions: Consume leafy green vegetables, fruit juice, and plenty of water. Avoid sugar, candies, and all sweets. Avoid straining the bowels. Establish habit of going to toilet at regular times.

FORMULA 1

5 teaspoons minced dried dates
5 teaspoons almond, mashed into a pulp
10 teaspoons honey

Preparation: Grind the first two ingredients separately, combine, and add honey.
Dosage: 3 teaspoons twice daily.

Note: This formula also useful for hemorrhoids and chronic constipation.

FORMULA 2

1 teaspoon senna leaves
1 teaspoon ground ginger (dried or fresh)
1 teaspoon fennel seeds
1 teaspoon rock salt

Preparation: Make a fine powder of all ingredients.
Dosage: 1 teaspoon with water at bedtime.

COUGH

FORMULA 1

1 cup ginger water
2 teaspoons honey

Preparation: Mix ingredients together.
Dosage: Two or three times per day.

FORMULA 2

2 teaspoons poppy seed
3 teaspoons cut licorice root

Preparation: Boil in 1 cup water for ten minutes and strain.
Dosage: Twice daily.

OTHER

Use Formula 2 under Asthma heading.

Dosage: 1 teaspoon, three or four times daily.

DIABETES

Frequent and excessive urination, excessive thirst, weak appetite, and general debility are common signs. Sugar is present in the blood and urine. The presence and amount of sugar in the urine should be determined by a test administered by a physician.

Instructions: Avoid sweets and sweet fruits. Avoid such carbohydrates as white potato, sweet potato, and rice. Mild exercise is advised.

FORMULA 1

8 teaspoons crushed cumin seeds

Preparation: Make a fine powder.
Dosage: 1/2 teaspoon, with water, twice daily.

DIARRHEA

Instructions: Eat a light diet. Avoid chili peppers and spicy foods.

FORMULA 1

1 teaspoon powdered ginger
1 teaspoon powdered cumin
1 teaspoon powdered cinnamon

Preparation: Combine all three powders, add honey, and mix into a thick paste.
Dosage: 1/2 to 1 teaspoon, three times daily.

FORMULA 2

3 teaspoons powdered ginger
5 teaspoons fennel seed
honey, as needed

Preparation: Grind ginger and fennel into a powder. Add honey to make thick paste.
Dosage: 1 teaspoon in tea, three times daily and before bedtime.

FORMULA 3

6 ounces Madjool dates
3 teaspoons myrrh
rose water, as needed

Preparation: Make a fine powder of first two ingredients, then mix with rose water to moisten. Make fingernail-sized pills.
Dosage: Two pills, twice daily.

DYSENTERY

Frequent bowel movements, sometimes mixed with mucus and blood, gripping pain, and pain in abdomen.
Instructions: A diet of yogurt and rice is advised.

FORMULA 1

10 pomegranate flowers

Preparation: Grind flowers with 1/2 teacup water. Strain.
Dosage: Twice daily.

FORMULA 2

2 teaspoons green leaves of rose bush

Preparation: Grind with 1/2 teacup of water. Strain.
Dosage: Twice daily.

HEADACHE

Headache is of different types, sometimes felt in different parts, or all over the head. Nausea and vomiting may also be present.

FORMULA 1

3 teaspoons lavender flowers
3 teaspoons coriander seeds
5 black peppercorns

Preparation: Grind all ingredients into fine powder.
Dosage: Take one-half of dose with water, early in the morning, then rest in bed for thirty minutes.

FORMULA 2

1 teaspoon Spanish saffron
1 teaspoon gum myrrh
1 teaspoon cinnamon

Preparation: Make a fine powder of all ingredients, add a little water, and mix well into a paste.
Administration: Put the paste onto a piece of clean cotton cloth, and apply to one or both temples.

FORMULA 3

6 teaspoons jasmine water
½ teaspoon sea salt

Preparation: Dissolve the salt in the jasmine water and preserve in a clean glass dropper bottle.
Dosage: Two drops in each nostril, twice a day or as needed.

FORMULA 4
(for migraine)

1/2 teaspoon black mustard seeds

Preparation: Grind with 3 tablespoons water and strain.
Dosage: One or two drops in nostrils.

HEMORRHOIDS

Constipation, passing of hard stool with blood, burning and irritation in anus, and discomfort in sitting. Presence of pile mass in anus. Blood may ooze out after bowel movement.

Instructions: Exercise lightly. Light diet with green vegetables is advised. Avoid hot spices.

External Treatment: Rub anus with rose water or other flower water to soothe.

FORMULA 1

1 teaspoon henna leaves

Preparation: Grind henna leaves into powder with 1 cup water. Strain and let sit for twenty minutes.
Dosage: Drink 1/2 cup twice daily.

FORMULA 2

1/8 teaspoon coriander leaves
1/8 teaspoon red clay earth

Preparation: Grind to make a paste and apply to anus.

FORMULA 3

3 teaspoons marshmallow
3 teaspoons dill

Preparation: Put herbs inside a clean sterile cloth; wet with warm water.
Application: Apply to anal area for half-hour at a time.

INDIGESTION

Feeling of heaviness in stomach after eating. Lack of appetite, nausea, flatulence, and vomiting. This condition is usually due to faulty, irregular diet, especially eating before the previous meal is fully digested.

FORMULA 1

1 teaspoon fennel seeds
1 teaspoon cardamom seeds

Preparation: Make a fine powder of the seeds.
Dosage: 1/6 teaspoon with water twice daily after meals.

FORMULA 2

1 teaspoon fennel seed
1 teaspoon dried ginger
1 teaspoon cloves

Preparation: Grind fennel, ginger, and cloves into a fine powder. Add honey to make a thick paste. Preserve in a glass jar.
Dosage: 1 teaspoon fifteen minutes after each meal and at bedtime.

FORMULA 3

1 teaspoon rock salt
1/2 cup ginger water
1/2 cup lime water

Preparation: Mix, preserve in glass bottle, and expose to sun for three or four days.
Dosage: Mix 1 teaspoon with 1/2 cup of water. Take twice daily, after meals.

FORMULA 4

1–3 drops peppermint oil

Preparation: Mix 1–3 drops of peppermint oil with 8 ounces water.
Dosage: Drink as needed.

INFLAMMATION OF GUMS AND TOOTHACHE

Swollen, reddened, painful gums. Person may become restless and agitated because of toothache.

FORMULA 1

1 cup ginger water
1/2 teaspoon salt

Preparation: Mix salt with ginger water.
Administration: Apply by dipping finger in water and rubbing on gums.

FORMULA 2

Oil of clove, as needed

Administration: Apply to gums or aching tooth.

FORMULA 3

3 teaspoons vinegar
6 teaspoons rose water

Preparation: Mix vinegar and rose water in glass.
Administration: Gargle with solution three times per day.

JAUNDICE

The color of urine and eyes is yellow. Skin is pale. Stools may be white or grayish. Generally nausea, vomiting, fever, and weakness.

FORMULA 1

1 teaspoon henna leaves

Preparation: Crush leaves, boil in 1 1/2 cups water, strain.
Dosage: Take as such in the morning.

FORMULA 2

1 teaspoon roasted chickory root

Preparation: Soak in 1 cup water overnight; strain in morning.
Dosage: Drink whole cup in morning.

FORMULA 3

1 teaspoon chickory seeds
1 teaspoon cut licorice root
1 teaspoon rock salt

Preparation: Make a fine powder of all ingredients.
Dosage: 1/2 teaspoon with water twice daily.

LOSS OF HAIR

FORMULA

2 cups roots of fig tree
1 quart coconut oil or olive oil

Preparation: Dry out fig roots in shade for three days. Then crush roots and immerse in oil for fifteen days. Strain and preserve in glass bottle.
Administration: Massage on scalp at bedtime. Leave on overnight.

OBESITY

FORMULA 1
(to curb excessive appetite)

1 teaspoon valerian root
1 teaspoon nutmeg

Preparation: Grind the two herbs into fine powder.
Dosage: 1/6 teaspoon, thirty minutes before meals, with water.

FORMULA 2

1 teaspoon lime juice

Dosage: Take with 1 cup water in the morning on an empty stomach.

PAINFUL MENSTRUATION

This condition is preceded by severe pain in the thighs, pubic region, and groin. Sometimes heavy nausea and vomiting occur. Usually blood flow is very scanty.

FORMULA 1

1 teaspoon gum myrrh
1 teaspoon juniper berries

Preparation: Boil in 1 cup of water. Strain.
Dosage: Take in morning for seven to ten days after menstrual period has ended.

FORMULA 2

1 3/4 teaspoons powdered rhubarb

Preparation: Dehydrate and make into a fine powder.
Dosage: 1/8 teaspoon of rhubarb powder with water twice daily, for one to two weeks following end of period.

FORMULA 3

1 teaspoon fennel seeds
1 teaspoon wild rue
1 teaspoon wormwood
1 teaspoon rose hips
1 teaspoon chopped figs
4 teaspoons honey

Preparation: Boil all ingredients in 1 cup water for five minutes. Strain and preserve.
Dosage: Consume in tablespoon doses twice a day for three days. Stop for three days. Then repeat dose.

SKIN ULCERS AND BOILS

FORMULA 1

Linseed as needed

Preparation: Grind with water to make a paste.
Administration: Apply to boil (which, after it is drawn out, should be lanced).

SLEEPLESSNESS

FORMULA 1

1/2 teaspoon poppy seeds
1/2 teaspoon lettuce seeds

Preparation: Boil in 1 cup water, strain, and sweeten with honey.
Dosage: Twice daily.

FORMULA 2

1/2 teaspoon cinnamon stick

Preparation: Boil in 1 cup water for five minutes, strain, and sweeten with honey.
Dosage: Twice daily.

FORMULA 3

3 drops rose oil
3 drops violet oil
1 ounce sweet almond oil

Preparation: Thoroughly mix the three oils and preserve.
Administration: Apply to scalp, ears and soles of feet before retiring. A small amount can be applied to the anus as well.

VAGINAL ITCHING

Itching and burning in vagina; burning sensation while urinating. Restlessness.

Instructions: Avoid close, tight-fitting underwear, especially made of nylon or other synthetic fabrics. Acute cleanliness of the vaginal area is required. Bathe immediately after urinating and after sexual intercourse.

FORMULA 1

3 teaspoons fennel seeds
2 teaspoons lily-of-the-valley root
1/2 teaspoon pomegranate flowers
1/2 teaspoon rosehips

Preparation: Pound and grind into powder. Sift.
Dosage: 1 to 2 teaspoons daily with buttermilk or a glass of juiced green grapes.

FORMULA 2

1/3 teaspoon camphor herb
6 teaspoons rose water

Preparation: Grind camphor in rose water.
Administration: Soak a tampon in solution and apply to vagina for thirty minutes. Repeat as necessary.

8

Fasting: The Best Medicine

Every act of the son of Adam is for him except fasting. It is done for My sake, and I will give as much reward for it as I like.

Allah, the Majestic and the Exalted

Fasting is the oldest known form of natural healing. The methods employed range from discontinuance of a single food for a short period of time, up through total abstinence from all foods and liquids for extended periods.

For many people who have never fasted, the idea seems strange, and some even consider it quite dangerous. These conceptions are not utterly unfounded, because incorrectly applied fasting can result in severe disorders of the body, and even death.

Correctly observed fasts are adjusted according to the cycles of the moon and other planets, as well as many other phenomena. Fasting is actually the epitome of a natural way of life, and its benefits do not end at the correction of the body and restoration of health.

Before taking up any kind of fast, it is important to understand the rationale for fasting. Most Westerners who fast do so to cleanse the body and improve health. However, these are incorrect intentions with which to begin a fast.

The Sufis probably have more experience than any other group of humans in performing fasts. The accounts are legion of Sufi shaykhs and disciples who endured fasts of varying durations, frequently with miraculous results. As has been noted, the Sufi does not take up any physical procedure relating to health for any reason except to earn the pleasure of the Most High God. Allah has informed us in the Holy Qur'an: "O ye who believe! Prescribed unto you is fasting even as it was prescribed unto those before you, that perhaps you may become God-conscious" (2:183).

All of the creation, except man, follows the dictates of God derived from natural laws. Animals do not have to be restrained from overeating and dietary abuses. But for humans, the love of material life and the temptations of the physical desires are responsible for the vast majority of illnesses. Therefore, Allah the Most Kind has provided guidance to control and annul these appetites by the mechanism of the fast.

The Qur'an states that a human cannot attain salvation unless the low desires are restrained: "And as for him who fears to stand before his Lord and restrains himself from low desires, the paradise is surely the abode" (79:40–41).

The exercise of abstaining from things that are ordinarily lawful and permitted in life, solely for the sake of Allah, strengthens morality and self-control and deepens awareness of Allah. This is what distinguishes fasting in Islam and Sufism from ordinary fasting for health.

The primary fast to be taken up is that generally called Ramaḍan in Islam. Ramaḍan is one of the months of the Islamic calendar (see Appendix I for Islamic months)—the month during which the Qur'an, as well as the Torah, the Psalms of David, and the New Testament, all were first sent down from Allah.

The excellence of fasting is known from these two statements of the Prophet (s.a.w.s.).

> By the one in whose hand is my life, the fragrance of the mouth of a fasting man is dearer to Allah than the fragrance of musk.

> Paradise has a gate named Rayyān. None except a fasting person will enter Paradise by that gate.

Allah has promised a vision of Him as reward for fasting.

The word *ramaḍan* does not actually mean "fast." The technical term for fasting is *ṣiyām*, whose root word means "to be at rest." By abstaining from food, drink, and sexual intercourse, these functions of the body are granted rest, and an opportunity to become revivified.

The general fast during the month of Ramaḍan is enjoined upon the whole humanity; those who actually do it are Muslims. Many persons who have close contact with Muslims also engage in this form of fast and derive some of the benefits from it. But there are several regulations which must be followed for any fast to be valid.

First, one must clearly state the intention to fast. Since Allah has said that we will be judged according to our intentions, one cannot get the benefits of good actions which occur entirely by accident. For example, if one was deprived of food by being lost in the wilderness, this would not constitute a formal fast, because one would have eaten if the opportunity were present. This formal declaration to perform an action is termed *niyyat*. It is preferably stated in Arabic, but is just as valid in any language. One may simply state: "I intend to offer fast this day, for the sake of Allah and only for the sake of Allah."

Having entered into this formal pledge with Allah, having made this promise, if one intentionally breaks the fast during the avowed period, one is liable to compensate for the fast by making up one or more days.

Generally, to perform a fast day the following conditions must all be met:

1. The *niyyat*, or intention to fast, must be made, aloud or silently.
2. The period of the fast must extend from the time just before sunrise (*fajr*) until just after sunset (*maghrib*).*
3. During the period of the fast, total abstinence from the following is required: food, drink (including water), smoking or consumption of tobacco, sexual intercourse, and any form of negativity, backbiting, fighting, cursing, arguing, and similar behaviors.
4. Semen may not be deliberately emitted, nor may one deliberately vomit.
5. Pregnant or lactating women, the seriously ill, the aged, and the insane are exempted from fasting, but in some cases may be liable to make up missed days. A woman does not fast on days when she is menstruating, but must make up the missed days. When her period ends, she must resume fasting. Children under the age of twelve generally are excluded from the fast, but may fast part of the day or for some of the days.
6. The fast is broken after sunset with a date or a glass of water, followed by a modest meal.

There are several dozens of special cases which apply to the fasting man or woman, and the advice of a practicing Muslim shaykh should be sought to resolve any question.

The special nature of fasting is that it engenders forbearance and sacrifice. Fasting occurs in the mind primarily, and so it is hidden from all human eyes, visible only to the Eye of God: it is a secret action.

During the time from midnight to the beginning of the fast, it was the practice of the Prophet (s.a.w.s.) to eat a meal, called *saḥūr*. This may consist of any lawful foods. The fast is usually broken by eating one or a few dates, followed by some water, which must be done prior to offering the sunset (*maghrib*) prayer. Even though cleaning the teeth is permitted, it is more meritorious if one does not do so after midday.

In addition to these injunctions, one should be engaged as much as possible in reading and reciting the Holy Qur'an, and should distribute as much charity as one is capable of.

*See Chapter 9, "Ṣalāt," for computing sunrise and sunset correctly.

Such are the minimum regulations for fasting. It is the fast of the general people, and entered into for the purpose of restraining oneself from eating and drinking and sexual passions. A higher form of the fast consists of (in addition to the above) refraining from wrong actions of hands, feet, sight, and other limbs or organs of the body.

The saints perform the very greatest kind of fast, a fast of the mind. In other words, these people do not think of anything except Allah. They consider their existence in this world only as a seed for growth into the next world. This fast also includes restraining the eyes from any evil sight, and shunning useless talk, falsity, slander, obscenity, and hypocrisy. In short, the fasters keep silent, and when they do speak, it is only to remember God. This fast is so strict that one cannot even listen to forbidden speech coming from others. One must leave the presence of the person who violates these prohibitions.

Moreover, the Sufis, when they do break the fast, eat only the minimum amount required to stem hunger. The correct meal following this fast is the one being eaten by the poorest people in one's community.

In addition to the obligatory fast of the sacred month, the Sufis engage in various optional fasts, which are called *nafil* fasts. Some of these occur every year, some every month, and some every week. The accompanying list summarizes the entire spectrum of fasts engaged in by the Sufis.

Although the main intention and desired effects of fasting occur in the realm of the soul and its evolution, it nonetheless remains a fact that most people achieve physical results of the fast as well.

As discussed earlier, disease frequently is attributed to incomplete digestion of the nutrients at one or more stages of digestion. During a fast, the ordinary work performed in the digestion of foods is reduced, thereby allowing the body to eliminate superfluous matters and to repair damage done by long-term dietary abuses.

When this occurs, the body responds in special ways. The first action the body takes, when given the opportunity, is to generate the strange heat of fever. This special kind of heat causes a very rapid processing ("cooking" down) of the excess matters, regardless of what they may be. The substances are thus refined into a form which can be eliminated by the body. The elimination occurs in one (and sometimes more) of five ways, which are called the five forms of healing crisis: nosebleed, vomiting, diarrhea, perspiration, and urination.

By saying that this elimination occurs in a healing crisis, I mean that the body is putting out the excess, frequently harmful and toxic by-products of abnormal, incomplete digestion. A healing crisis by urination is not the same thing as normal urination. The volume and frequency may be as high as five or more times an hour for several hours. A healing crisis by diarrhea could consist of fifteen or more motions in several hours.

FAST DAYS OF THE SUFIS

Ramaḍan: The thirty-day fast obligatory upon all Muslims.

Other Annual Fasts: The days of ᶜArafāt (during the month of Dhul-Hijjah); the days of ᶜArshurah; the first ten days of Dhul-Hijjah; the first ten days of the month of Moharram; and as much of the month of Shaᶜbān as possible. (Note: It is not permitted to fast the three days prior to the beginning of Ramaḍan, nor the feast days of ᶜĪd al-Fitr and ᶜĪd al-Aḍḥā).

Monthly Fasts: The best days to keep fast during any month are the first day, the middle day, and the last day of every month. In addition, there is fasting on the *ayyām bayād*—the thirteenth, fourteenth, and fifteenth days of the moon's cycle.

Weekly Fasts: While fasting any week, one should endeavor to fast Thursday, Friday, and Monday, which are the days of excellence.

Daily Fasts: The Prophet (s.a.w.s.) forbade fasting every day. The best way to maintain maximum fasting is to fast every other day. The Prophet (s.a.w.s.) said, "The treasures of the world were presented to me. I rejected them and said: I shall remain hungry for one day and take food on the next. When I take food I shall praise Thee, and when I remain hungry I shall seek humility from Thee." And then he said: "There is no better fast than this."

Oddly enough, these healing crises are precisely the events that Western medicine labels as illness and disease. Consequently, the efforts to arbitrarily block or end these normal eliminative functions cut short the most effective inherent health-building mechanisms the body possesses!

The forms of healing crisis are mentioned because during fasting—especially for one who has never taken it up before—one or more of these are likely to transpire after the third or fourth days (sometimes even within a few hours). A pounding headache, perhaps a slightly elevated temperature or fever, sweating, and similar signs show that the body is moving into a corrective mode. When the diarrhea or vomiting begins, one who is unacquainted with the benefits and effects of fasting may conclude that he has contracted the flu or a respiratory problem, having become "weakened" by fasting!

Many people are unwilling to endure any discomfort or unpleasantness whatsoever, and thus resort to various chemical drugs, which will unfortunately put an immediate end to any healing actions of the body. This may suffice to get a person back to work, or prop him or her up to attend an important function; but over years and years of suppressing these eliminations, the toxic matters back up within the system, until organ damage occurs and there is no hope for a cure, except by the most drastic means. Even then it is difficult and gruesome.

Effort and discipline are required to make it through these recommended fasts. I suggest persons with no experience begin with just one day, or part of a day, and gradually extend it to the desired level of performance. Muslims have a special advantage, for they are strengthened and helped by Allah to complete a full thirty days each year. One of the great Sufis was said to have fasted on alternate days during the last forty years of his life. And, at that, when he did eat, if he discovered he was deriving any pleasure from the food, he would immediately spit it out half-chewed. He lived to be ninety-six years old.

Allah the Almighty has promised uncountable rewards for those who fast. One such reward for the fortunate ones occurs during the last ten days of Ramaḍān. This is known as Laylat al-Qadr (Night of Power). For one who has performed the fast perfectly and according to the strictest criteria, Allah sends an angel to personally meet this person, and any wish whatsoever the person may make is granted. *Yā Ḥayyu! Ya Qāyyūm!*

Fasting is prescribed by the Most High God as a great blessing upon His humanity. As the Maker of human bodies, He knows the best techniques and practices for maintaining its health. And not only is fasting the best and safest means of protecting the physical health, but it also carries immense spiritual rewards.

One other aspect of physical life bears significantly upon human health. It is the cornerstone of all Sufi activities, the *ṣalāt*, which serves as the ladder by which one may approach God.

9

Ṣalāt: The Postures of the Prophets

The Great and Glorious God does not insist upon the performance of any other devotion as much as He does on the performance of ṣalāt.

Hazrat Khwāja Gharib Nawāz (r.a.)

Sūrat al-Fātiḥah, the Opening of the Holy Qur'an, is in one sense the most condensed and concentrated prayer one can utter. It is said that the whole of the Qur'an is encapsulated in this opening *sūrah*. Two of its verses are a special imploring by the servant to God Almighty for His guidance:

Ihdīnāṣ-ṣirāṭ al-mustaqīm
Ṣirāṭ alladhīna an^{c}amta ^{c}alayhim.

Show us the straight path,
The path of those whom You love and have favored.

Not only as the Most Kind God provided humans with the best possible invocation to Him, but immediately after He hears this sincere request, He informs His creatures of the means of attaining it—by revealing the entire Qur'an for the perfect and total guidance of humankind.

However, in the very first verses of the second *sūrah* of the Qur'an, Allah establishes the only keys that will open the blessings of this book:

Dhalikal-kitābu lā rayba fīh
Hudā lil-muttaqīn;
Alladhinā yu'minūna bil-ghaybi
wa yuqīmūnaṣ-ṣalāta wa mimmā
razaqnāhum yunfiqūn.

This is the Scripture
wherein there is no doubt,
A guidance to those who shun evil,
Who believe in the Unseen,
and establish *ṣalāt*, and
spend of that which We
have bestowed upon them.

The word *ṣalāt* in Arabic is translated as prayer or worship, and also supplications for forgiveness, compassion, and mercy. (In Persian, Turkish, and Urdu, the term is *namāz*.)

Western scholars have unfortunately misrepresented the true conception of *ṣalāt* by translating the word simply as "prayer" or "worship." In fact, the practice of *ṣalāt* is very specific and forms the most unique and central feature of religious life in Islam and Sufism. The Holy Prophet Muhammad (s.a.w.s.) is reported to have said, "The difference between a believer in God and a disbeliever in Him is the performance of *ṣalāt*."

The great saint Hazrat Khwāja Gharib Nawāz (r.a.) commented on the importance of the *ṣalāt* with the following statements:

> Without performing *ṣalāt*, none can approach God, because *ṣalāt* is the climax in the process of such approach for the pious.
>
> *Ṣalāt* is the ladder leading to the proximity [*qurb*] of God.
>
> *Ṣalāt* is a trust committed to human care by Almighty God, a secret relationship existing between the worshiper and the Worshiped.

The Indian mystic musician Hazrat Inayat Khan, who brought some Sufi ideas to the West in the early part of this century, said, "A person who never accomplishes [*ṣalāt*] has no hope of ever advancing any other way, for every posture has a wonderful meaning and a particular effect . . . it is to be prescribed before further sacred teachings. If he fails to advance in this, there is no hope for his future."

Ṣalāt is at once an external and an internal practice: a set of physical exercises (some have compared them to yoga *asanas*), and the richest spiritual nourishment. By considering each of these aspects in some detail, we can learn why the Sufis have considered in many cases that they would rather die than forgo their *ṣalāt*. *Mā shā' Allāh!*

The practice of *ṣalāt* is performed at five regular intervals throughout the day as a minimum and can be done at other times according to the capacities of the worshiper. The times of performance are fixed according to the journey of the sun and planets across the heavens. These times are as follows:

Fajr: Begins approximately forty-five minutes before sunrise and extends up to the rising of the sun.

***Ẓuhr*:** Begins after the sun has passed the median point in the sky and has just begun its downward arc.

***ᶜAṣr*:** Begins when the sun has crossed a bisection of the arc made by the sun, midpoint between noon and the line of the horizon; or when the body's shadow is equal to two body lengths.

***Maghrib*:** Begins just after the sun has set below the horizon and no light is left reflecting off the clouds (i.e., there is no more redness).

***ᶜIshā*:** Begins when night has fully fallen, approximately one hour and twenty minutes after the time of *maghrib*, or sunset.

By following these prayer times, one is perfectly attuned to the motions of the planets, seasonal changes, and geographic variations. In so doing, one becomes harmonized with all of the natural cycles of the universe.

There are three aspects to the *ṣalāt*: thought, word, and action. Before beginning the *ṣalāt*, one must clean oneself of any physical dirt on the body or clothing, or on the place where one intends to pray. At this same time, one must drive out all negative or evil thoughts and cleanse the mind to concentrate fully upon the glory of Allah the Almighty. This preparation, called *wuḍū'*, consists of washing the hands, rinsing the mouth (and brushing teeth if necessary), snuffing water up the nose, wiping the face from brow to chin and from ear to ear, washing the forearms from the wrists up to the elbows, wiping over the head and the back of the neck, and, finally, washing the feet up to the ankle bone. Each of these washings is repeated three times and must be done in the sequence described.

When these actions have been carefully completed, one goes to the place of prayer and, assuming a humble attitude, with head down, hands at sides, and feet evenly spaced below the shoulders, utters the intention to offer the *ṣalāt*, as follows:

> I intend to offer [the obligatory number of] *raᶜkat*s of *ṣalāt*, and face the *qiblah*, the Exalted Kaᶜbah, for the sake of Allah and Allah alone. I take refuge with Allah from the rejected and evil satan, and I begin in the Name of Allah, Most Gracious, Most Merciful.

This invocation may be made in Arabic, but any language will suffice as well. However, the remainder of the *ṣalāt* must be recited entirely in Arabic. (Later chapters discuss the Arabic vowels, sounds, and breath patterns.) The one offering prayer must be facing in the direction of the city of Mecca, Saudi Arabia. (In the United States, this would mean facing generally eastward.)

The *ṣalāt* is done by assuming eight separate positions of the body (*arkān*), and reciting various Qur'anic verses with each posture. These postures are illustrated in turn, and a brief description is given of the benefits ascribed to each.

POSTURE 1

Bring hands, palms open, up to ears, and place thumbs behind earlobes, as *"Allāhu akbar"* (God is Great) is uttered.

Name of Posture: Niyyat
Time to Be Held: 5 seconds
Recitation: Allāhu akbar.

Beneficial Effects: Body feels relieved of weight owing to even distribution on both feet. Straightening back improves posture. Mind is brought under control of intellect. Vision is sharpened by focusing upon floor, where head will prostrate. Muscles of upper and lower back are loosened. Higher and lower centers of brain are united to form singleness of purpose.

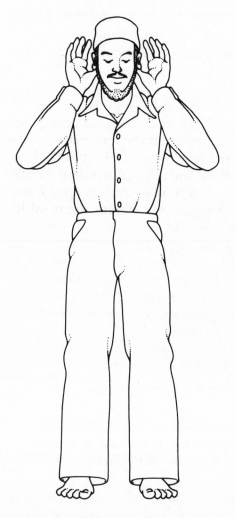

POSTURE 2

Place hands, right over left, just below navel.

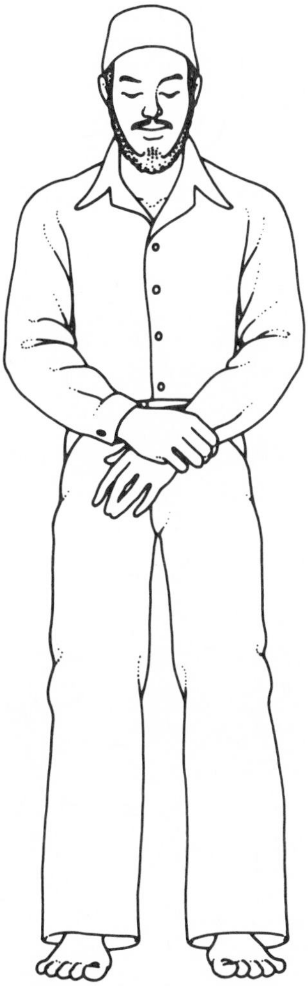

Name of Posture: Qiyām
Duration: 40–60 seconds
Recitation:
Bismi Llāh ir-Raḥmān ir-Raḥīm
Al-ḥamdu li-Llāhi rabb il-ᶜālamīn.
Ar-Raḥmān, ir-Raḥīm.
Māliki yawm id-Dīn.
Iyyāka na ᶜbudu wa iyyāka nasta ᶜīn.
Ihdināṣ-ṣirāṭ al-mustaqīm.
Ṣirāṭ alladhīna anᶜamta ᶜalayhīm
Ghayril-maghḍūbi ᶜalayhīm wa lāḍ-ḍālīn.
Āmīn.

(In the Name of Allah, the Beneficent,
the Merciful.
All praise be to Allah, Lord of the Worlds.
The Beneficent, the Merciful.
Master of the Day of Judgment.
Thee only do we worship.
Thee alone we ask for help.
Show us the straight path.
The path of those whom You love and favor,
Not the path of those who have earned
Thine anger, nor are leading astray.
Be it so.)

Following these words, a short chapter of at least three verses should be recited from the Holy Qur'an (see Appendix II for suitable examples).

Beneficial Effects: Extends concentration, causes further relaxation of legs and back, generates feelings of humility, modesty, and piety. In the recital of the above verses, virtually all of the sounds that occur in Arabic are uttered, stimulating dispersal of all of the ninety-nine divine attributes in perfectly controlled degrees throughout the body, mind, and soul. The sound vibrations of the long vowels *ā*, *ī*, and *ū* stimulate the heart, thyroid, pineal gland, pituitary, adrenal glands, and lungs, purifying and uplifting them all.

POSTURE 3

Bend at waist, placing palms on knees with fingers spread. Back is parallel to ground, such that if a glass of water were on the back, it would not spill. Eyes are looking down, directly ahead. Do not bend the knees.

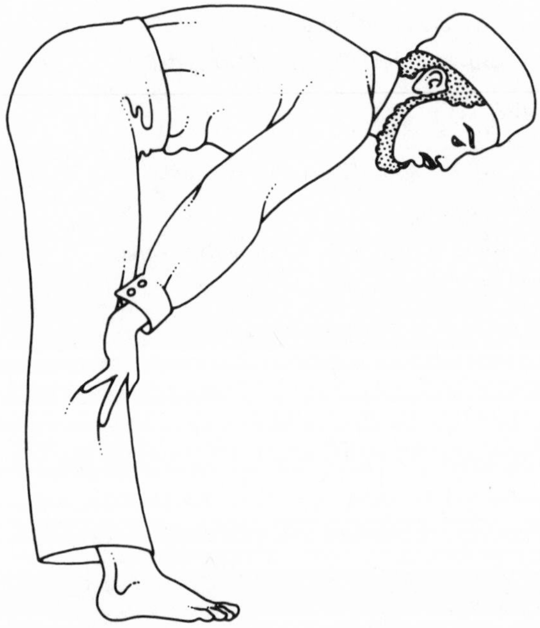

Name: Rukū^{c}
Duration: 12 seconds
Recitation: While bending at the waist, recite Allāhu akbar, *then:*
Subḥāna Rabbī al-^{c}Aẓīm
Subḥāna Rabbī al-^{c}Aẓīm
Subḥāna Rabbī al-^{c}Aẓīm

(Holy is my Lord, the Magnificent)

Beneficial Effects: Fully stretches the muscles of the lower back, thighs, and calves. Blood is pumped into upper torso. Tones muscles of stomach, abdomen, and kidneys. Over time, this posture improves the personality, generating sweet kindness and inner harmony.

POSTURE 4

While rising from the bending position of *ruku^c*, recite *Sami^{c}a Llāhu li-man ḥamidah. Rabbanā wa lakal-ḥamd* (Allah hears the one who praises Him; Our Lord, Yours is the praise). Then return to standing position, arms at side.

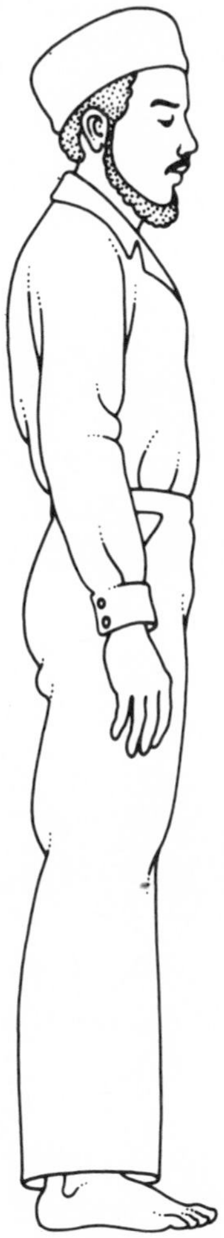

Name: Qauma

Duration: 6 seconds

Recitation: After holding for six seconds, say:

Allāhu akbar

and move to next position.

Beneficial Effects: The fresh blood moved up into torso in previous posture returns to its original state, carrying away toxins. Body regains relaxation and releases tension.

POSTURE 5

Place both hands on knees and lower yourself slowly and easily into a kneeling position. Then touch the head and hands to the ground. The following seven body parts should be in contact with the ground: forehead, two palms, two knees, toes of both feet. The end position of this posture is given below.

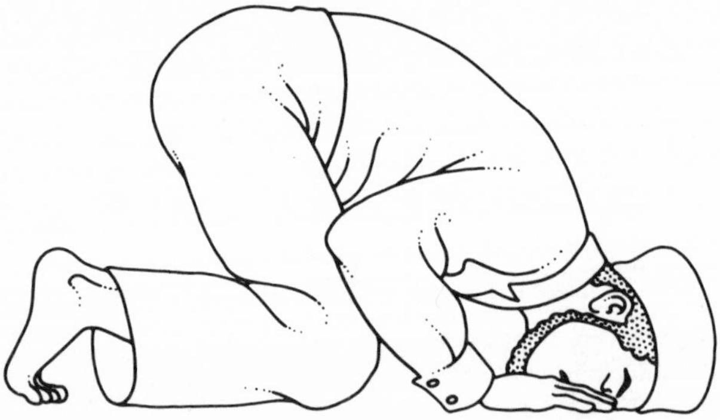

Name: Sajdah
Duration: 12 seconds
Recitation:
Subḥāna Rabbī al-^{c}Alā
Subḥāna Rabbī al-^{c}Alā
Subḥāna Rabbī al-^{c}lā

(Glory be to my Lord, the Most Supreme)

Beneficial Effects: Knees forming a right angle allow stomach muscles to develop and prevents growth of flabbiness in midsection. Increases flow of blood into upper regions of body, especially the head (including eyes, ears, and nose) and lungs; allows mental toxins to be cleansed by blood. Maintains proper position of fetus in pregnant women. Reduces high blood pressure. Increases elasticity of joints. Annihilates egotism and vanity. Increases patience and reliance upon God. Increases spiritual stations and produces high psychic energy throughout body. This posture of supreme submission and humility is the essence of worship.

POSTURE 6

Reciting *Allāhu akbar*, rise from Position 5 and assume the sitting posture shown here.

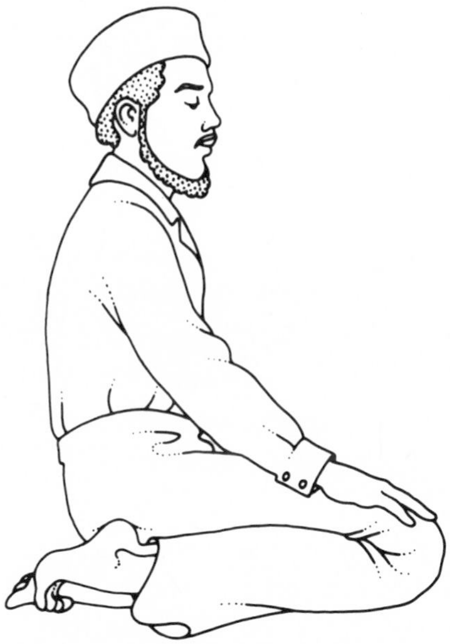

Name: Quᶜūd
Duration: 6 seconds
Recitation: At end of 6 seconds, recite Allāhu akbar *and repeat actions of Position 5 exactly.*

Beneficial Effects: For men, the heel of the right foot is curled up and the weight of the leg and part of the body rests upon it. This aids detoxification of the liver and stimulates peristaltic action of the large intestine. Women keep both feet, soles up, underneath their bodies. The body returns to even greater relaxation, and the posture assists digestion by forcing the contents of the stomach downward.

POSTURE 7

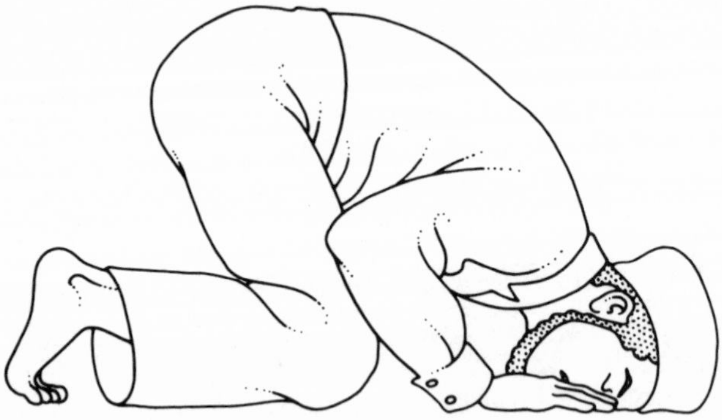

Repeat motions of Posture 5 exactly. Then, reciting Allāhu akbar, *return to sitting as in Posture 6.*

Beneficial Effects: Repetition of the deep prostration within a few seconds cleanses the respiratory, circulatory, and nervous systems. Gives experience of lightness of body and emotional happiness. Oxygenation of entire body is accomplished. Balances sympathetic and parasympathetic nervous systems.

POSTURE 8

From Posture 5, with head in prostration, lift the head away from the floor and bring the torso backward. Placing hands on knees, reverse the procedure for going down, and, while again reciting *Allāhu akbar*, return to the standing position. This completes one *raᶜkat* of prayer.

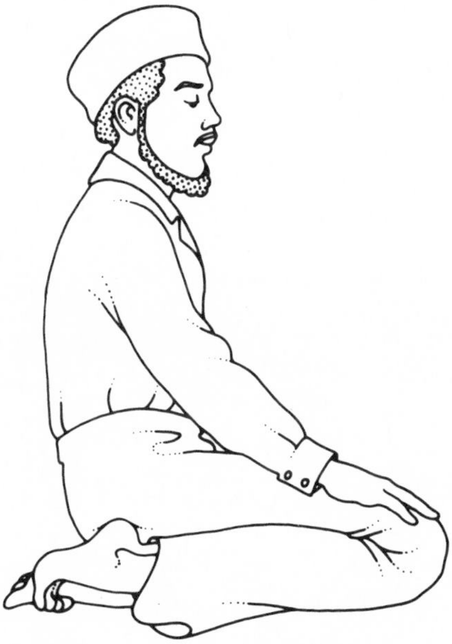

The *ṣalāt* is done in either two, three, or four *ra^{c}kats*, according to the time of day:

Fajr:	*2 ra^{c}kats*
Ẓuhr:	*4 ra^{c}kats*
^{c}Asr:	*4 ra^{c}kats*
Maghrib:	*3 ra^{c}kats*
Isha:	*4 ra^{c}kats*

At the end of each two units of prayer, the following supplication is added:

At-taḥiyyātu li-Llāhi waṣ-ṣalawātu waṭ-ṭayyibāt
As-salāmu 'alayka ayyuhān-Nabiyyu
Wa raḥmatu Llāhi wa barakātuhu
Was-salāmu ^{c}alaynā wa ^{c}alā ^{c}ibādi Llāhiṣ-ṣaliḥīn
Ash-hadu an lā ilāha illā Llāh
Wa ash-hadu anna Muḥammadan ^{c}abduhu wa rasūluh.

This supplication is recited as a re-creation of the celestial conversation which was held between Allah the Almighty and the Holy Prophet Muhammad (s.a.w.s.) during the night of the Heavenly Ascent (*Mi^{c}rāj*) of the Prophet. The lines were spoken as follows:

Muhammad: All greetings, blessings, and good acts are from You, my Lord.

Allah: Greetings to you, O Prophet, and the mercy and blessings of Allah.

Muhammad: Peace be unto us, and unto the righteous servants of Allah. I bear witness that there is no deity except Allah.

Allah: And I bear witness that Muhammad is His servant and messenger.

If the required number of *ra^{c}kat*s is but two, the *ṣalāt* would proceed to the next recitation. Otherwise, one or two more *ra^{c}kat*s are due. These are done exactly as the first two, except that no recitations occur after that of Sūrat al-Fātiḥah.

The recitations of the first two *ra^{c}kat*s are done aloud during the *ṣalāt* of *fajr* and *maghrib* and *^{c}isha*. At other times, all are recited silently.

When the proper number of two, three, or four *ra^{c}kat*s are completed, another prayer is said silently, praising and offering greetings and blessing upon the prophets and their families.

Allāhumma salli ^{c}alā sayyidinā Muḥammadin
wa ^{c}alā āli Muḥammadin
kama ṣallayta ^{c}alā Ibrāhīma
wa ^{c}alā āli Ibrāhīma
Innaka Ḥamīdun Majīd.
Allāhumma barik ^{c}alā Muḥammadin
wa ^{c}alā āli Muḥammadin
kamā barakta ^{c}alā Ibrāhīma
wa ^{c}alā āli Ibrāhīma.
Innaka Ḥamīdun Majīd.

(O Allah, bless our master Muhammad
and the family of Muhammad
as you have blessed Abraham
and the family of Abraham.
Surely You are the Praiseworthy, the Glorious.
O Allah, be gracious unto Muhammad
and unto the family of Muhammad
as You were gracious unto Abraham
and unto the family of Abraham.
Surely You are the Praiseworthy, the Glorious.)

At the end of this recitation, the head is hung low, then turned slowly to full extension to the right, so that the eyes can glance back over the shoulder, and one recites:

As-salāmu ^{c}alaykum wa raḥmatu Llāh

(Peace and blessings of God be upon you).

While turning the head to the left, one repeats the phrase:

As-salāmu ^{c}alaykum wa raḥmatu Llāh.

These last statements are addressed to the two recording angels, each of whom sits poised over the shoulder, recording respectively the good and wrongful actions. *Subḥān Allāh!*

Another interesting feature of the *ṣalāt* is that in the course of assuming three main positions (*qiyām, rukū^{c}*, and *sajdah*), one makes the physical shapes of the Arabic letters *alif, dal,* and *mim*. These letters spell the word *Adam*, the name of the first created human and the first prophet (a.s.). The illustrations on the following page show the body posture and letter correspondence.

The angels—who were created solely to worship Allah and do so as their natural behavior—perform all of these postures of worship. All the prophets of history (peace be upon them all) also used one or more of these postures. The prophet Muhammad (s.a.w.s.) was granted the grace of conveying to humanity the synthesis of all of the postures of all the prophets. *Al-ḥamdu li-Llāh il-Hayyūil-Qayyūm!*

Another important point regarding this practice, simply as a physical activity, is that persons of all ages can do it. It is smooth, flowing, and easy, and in time becomes the greatest physical development that is possible.

In the course of one day, the minimum performance consists of seventeen units of prayer, composed of nineteen separate positions during each *ra^{c}kat*. This is a total of 119 physical postures per day, or 3,570 postures monthly, or 42,840 postures yearly.

In the average adult lifetime of forty years, 1,713,600 postures are performed. Anyone so doing is protected and inoculated against a host of ailments and diseases, such as heart attack and other cardiac problems; emphysema; arthritis; bladder, kidney, and bowel problems; viral and bac-

SALAT POSTURES CORRESPONDING TO THE WORD ADAM

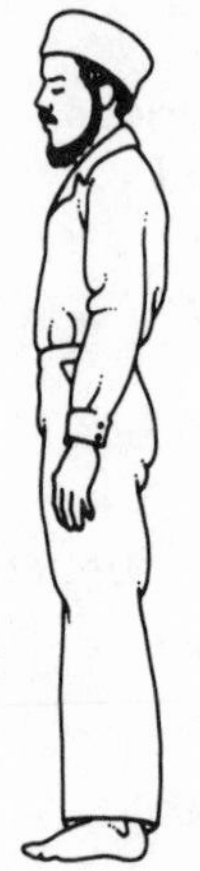

POSTURE OF QAUMA

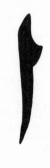

ا

LETTER ALIF (A)

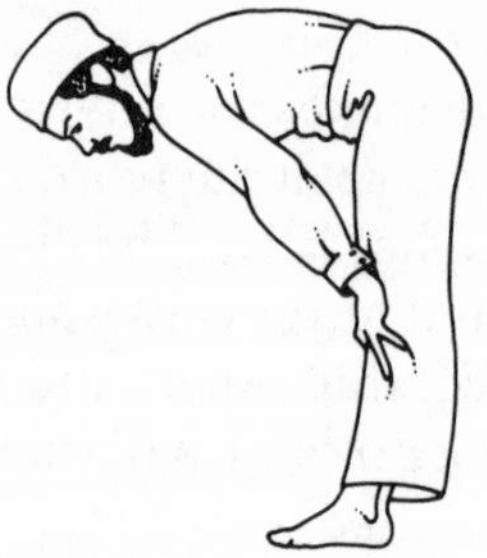

POSTURE OF RUKŪ

د

LETTER DAL (D)

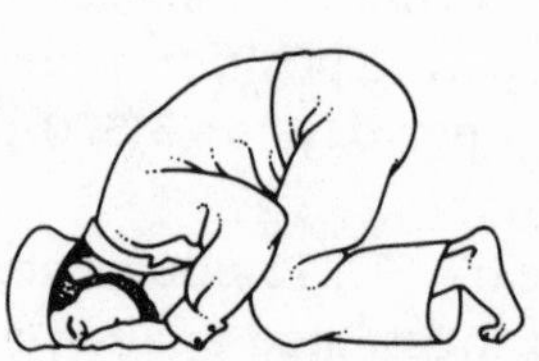

POSTURE OF SAJDAH

م

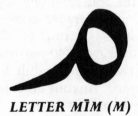

LETTER MĪM (M)

terial infections; eye diseases; loss of memory and senility; sciatica and spinal ailments; and many, many others. This practice can be done virtually anywhere, requires no special equipment, and costs nothing at all.

For the Sufis, the *ṣalāt* has even greater import in their lives because the carpet at the place of prayer becomes the stepping-off point for entering the divine reality, the *ḥaqīqat*.

The shaykhs generally state that there are four stages of practices for the aspirants to God: *sharīᶜat* (law), *ṭarīqat* (path), *ḥaqīqat* (truth), and *marᶜifat* (ecstasy).

The first requirement is to adopt and follow the *sharīᶜat*, the divine laws of human life, which in due course leads one onto the *ṣirāṭ al-mustaqīm*, the path. The enterprise of Sufism is frequently referred to as following *ṭarīqat*. This path leads one to the *ḥaqīqat*. Let me try to define this complex term. *Ḥaqīqat* is the final, incontrovertible and absolute truth of all existence. For example, some people believe God exists, some do not. Both cases cannot be true. The *ḥaqq* (or truth) of this matter is absolute. And we will all have this matter resolved with finality at the time of death. All hidden knowledge belongs to the realm of *ḥaqīqat*. When one attains this status of insight into the divine truths, there follows the stage called *maᶜrifat*—the overwhelming ecstasy of being a favored and chosen friend of the Beloved, Almighty God.

The performance of *ṣalāt* is required to attain any of these stations (which are sequential). But merely voicing sounds and standing in one place will not produce the desired effects. Several internal conditions must be present.

One must first of all approach the prayer with a sense of humility, with a recognition of the dependent position of the worshiper in relation to the Worshiped. Allah has informed us that we were "a thing unremembered, until I remembered you." There is not a single living person in the history of the world who was responsible for his or her own conception of life. Not only did we not exist: we did not even *know* that we did not exist!

We should put all thoughts except those of our merciful Creator out of our minds as we prepare to address Him. Worldly affairs must be shoved aside, with the understanding that the prayer is the means of stepping into the next world, of drawing near to God. If the mind is already filled with mundane thoughts, there will be no space for remembrance of God.

Another condition of prayer is that the meaning of the words uttered be as complete as possible. Even though they are spoken in Arabic, one should know the translated meanings in one's own language and should contemplate these meanings as deeply and sincerely as possible.

It is narrated in the Hadith that God said to Moses: "O Moses, when you want to remember Me, remember Me in such a way that your limbs tremble and that you hold Me dear at the time of remembrance and rest satisfied. When you stand before Me, stand before Me with a fearful mind like the poorest slave, and speak with Me with the tongue of a truthful man."

And then God revealed to him: "Tell your disobedient followers to remember Me. I took oath upon Myself that I shall remember one who remembers Me. When Abraham stood for prayer, the voice of his heart was heard from a distance of two miles. An individual will be forgiven in the next world according to the qualities of his mind, and not of his body."

Some people may wonder about the suggestion that we must fear God, asserting instead that we only need to think of God as kind and all-loving. A verse in the Holy Qur'an that makes this clear is found in Sūrat al-Baqarah (2:112):

Balā man aslama wajhahū li-Llahi
wa huwa muḥsinun
fa-lahū ajruhū ^{c}inda Rabbih
wa lā khawfun ^{c}alayhim
wa lā hum yaḥzanūn.

Nay, but whosoever gives up his own desires
while serving Allah and does good acts,
his reward is with his Lord;
They shall have no fears
And neither shall they grieve.

In other words, if one gives up one's own selfish desires and serves humanity solely for the sake of pleasing Allah, the reward is the totally and unrestricted protection, grace, and favor of Allah. When one has Allah, the Creator, Sustainer, and Ruler of the creation, as one's Protecting Friend, how could one ever be afraid or suffer sadness?

The ailments people experience in the *ṣalāt* are mainly concerned with distractions. These are both physical and mental. One is often distracted from deep concentration in prayer by room noises, conversations, muffled sounds from the street, and other goings-on. The medicine to correct this disease of *ṣalāt* is to cut off from the source of these distractions.

The Sufis find they can perform their divine services much better in dark, small, secluded rooms. If this is not possible, one must set apart a special place for worship and remembrance of Allah. Close the eyes, if necessary, because the eye is the first source of distraction.

The second cause of distraction is the mind itself: As each thought arises, it leads to another thought. In the early days of Islam, a camel driver came to Abū Bakr (r.a.), who was a very pious Muslim, and said, "I don't believe you can make two *ra^{c}kat*s of *ṣalāt* without thinking of something other than Allah." Abū Bakr asserted that he believed he could do it. The driver said that if Abū Bakr could perform two *ra^{c}kat*s without a single distracting thought, he would make him a gift of a camel, and he gestured to two camels nearby, one black and one brown.

Abū Bakr commenced his *ṣalāt*. When he finished, the camel driver looked at him anxiously. Abū Bakr, being a scrupulously honest man incapable of deception, confessed, "You were right, I couldn't make it through the *ṣalāt*. I was distracted." The camel driver was relieved that he had not lost a precious camel. Then the camel driver curiously asked, "But what was it that distracted you? What did you think about?" Abū Bakr answered, "I was trying to decide whether I would take the black camel or the brown one."

It is very difficult to cut the root of internal mental distractions. The best method is to concentrate as fully as possible on the meanings of what is being recited. If the mind does begin to wander, force it back to the Qur'anic meanings.

The Prophet (s.a.w.s.) recommended that one make *ṣalāt* in a room with no variegated colors, pictures, or extensive designs on the prayer carpet, and avoid wearing any kind of rings or other jewelry.

The Hadith state that when one stands in prayer, Allah lifts up the screen before Him, so that His servant faces him. The angels climb upon his two shoulders and pray in unison along with him and say *Āmīn* at the end of the prayer. Then they spread virtues out from the top of the worshiper's head to the end of the horizon. Then an angel proclaims: "If this servant had known Whom he had been invoking, he would not have looked around, distracted. The doors of heaven are thrown open for a praying person, and Allah takes pride before His angels for him, and the Face of God comes before his face." This opening of the doors to the Unseen is called *kashf*.

There are unfortunately some persons parading as pseudo-Sufis in the West, who foolishly assert that *ṣalāt* is unnecessary. They make the strange claim that such formal actions as *ṣalāt* are mere rituals, which the true spiritual aspirant can dispense with. Such misguided persons give the examples of Ibn ᶜArabī (r.a.), Mawlānā Rūmī (r.a.), Imam al-Ghazzalī (r.a.), and Manṣūr al-Ḥallāj (r.a.) as examples of truly liberated, free-thinking "Sufis." And they disdain anyone who makes *ṣalāt* or suggests its necessity as a backward-thinking "fundamentalist." I hope that the foregoing presentation of only some of the deeper aspects of the practice of *ṣalāt* will inspire people to learn and practice the *ṣalāt* to learn its truly marvelous effects. The great ones mentioned above, such as Rūmī and Ibn ᶜArabī, were in fact the most ardent and sincere followers of the *ṣalāt*.

One December in Konya, Mawlānā Rūmī (r.a.) had gone into his *ḥujrah* (meditation cell) to perform his nighttime prayers. When the time for the *fajr* (morning) prayer arrived, he did not appear. His followers became worried because in twenty years Mawlānā had never failed to join them in congregational prayer. As time passed and the *murīds'* alarm grew, someone finally decided to force the door open. Inside, they were startled to find the Mawlānā with his beard frozen to the ground, struggling to set himself free. In his supplications, he had begun weeping so copiously that a pool of tears had formed, and his prostration in the cold was so prolonged that the tears froze, trapping him by his beard!

Manṣūr al-Ḥallāj (r.a.) became famous in the history of Sufism for his alleged crime of offending the so-called orthodox clergy. However, he actually was tried and convicted on the charge of divulging divine secrets, which he had overheard while eavesdropping on his sister, who was a Sufi saint. The trial lasted over eight years. As Manṣūr al-Ḥallāj sat awaiting his execution during the last week of his life, he passed his time by punctually offering his *ṣalāt*, and on the last day of his life he performed 500 *ra*ᶜ*kat*s of *ṣalāt*!

The Sufis are the most strenuous supporters of *ṣalāt*. There is a story of Hazrat ᶜAbdul-Qādir Jīlānī (r.a.), who one morning was about to miss the time of the morning prayer. A cat came over to his side as he lay asleep and began nudging him until he awoke. Noticing the lateness of the time, ᶜAbdul-Qādir (r.a.) quickly offered his two *ra*ᶜ*kat*s of prayer. When he had finished, he looked at the cat, and with his spiritual insight, he saw that the cat was actually a satan. This puzzled the great saint, as to why a satan would wake him up for prayer. So he asked, "I can see you are a satan but why on earth did you wake me up for the *fajr* prayer?"

The cat answered, "You are just as pious and clever as my fellow satans said you were. Since you've discovered me, I might as well tell you. I knew that if you missed your obligatory prayer, you would have offered one hundred *ra*ᶜ*kat*s as compensation, so I woke you up so that you would only get the benefits of two."

In the course of Sufism, the shaykh assigned the *murīd* many practices that extend and enhance the basic practices of *ṣalāt*. First, added to the obligatory (*fard*) *ṣalāt*, are the extra prayers that the Prophet Muhammad (s.a.w.s.) used to do. These are called *sunnah*, and add several dozens more to the activities of worship of the *murīd*s. Later, the postures are held for varying periods—up to an hour or more—and verses from the Qur'an that are replete with mystical meaning are recited.

Ṣalāt is both the first and the final step for the true believer. It is the real means of uniting one with the whole of humanity, and with Almighty God. It is never altered in its essential features (and never has been for 1,400 years) and thus becomes the foundation upon which the more refined spiritual practices are built. For anyone who desires to enjoy the most excellent health, harmonizing the physical, mental, emotional, and spiritual life, there is no better medicine than the *ṣalāt*. As Hazrat Khwāja Gharib Nawāz frequently remarked to his followers: "Hurry up and perform the *ṣalāt*, before the Final Hour passes!"

It is incorrect to say, as some do, that when a seeker gains his desires, worship and devotion are no longer incumbent upon him; for the Chief of the World, blessings and peace of God be upon him, was always prostrating in worship and devotion before God. Although he had reached the summit of devotion, he would say, "O Lord, I am ashamed, for I did not worship You as I ought to have done."

The following chart provides the correct number of obligatory and optional *raᶜkat*s for the five daily prayers of *ṣalāt*.

NUMBER OF *RAᶜKATS* IN *ṢALĀT*					
Prayer	***Sunnah*** Before (Optional)	***Farḍ*** (Obligatory)	***Sunnah*** After (Optional)	***Nāfil*** (Optional)	***Witr*** (Highly Recommended)
Fajr (Recitation aloud)	2	2			
Zuhr (Silent)	4	4	2		
ᶜAṣr (Silent)	4	4			
Maghrib (First two *raᶜkat*s aloud)		3	2	2	
ᶜIshā (First two *raᶜkat*s aloud)	4	4	2	2	3

10

The Soul of the Rose

There are three things of this world that I have been made to prefer prayer, women, and scents.

Prophet Muhammad (s.a.w.s.)

The prophet Sulaymān (a.s.) was the one who first learned the healing properties of herbs and flowers. One day as he was standing for prayer in the mosque, a flower sprang up before him and said, "*As-salām ᶜalaykum*, Hazrat Sulaymān!" Hazrat Sulaymān returned the greeting and then asked, "What are you doing here? What are you for?" And the flower answered him that it was a remedy for such-and-such a disease. The next day, a different flower sprang up and told Hazrat Sulaymān the disease for which it was the remedy. Over a course of time, all of the medicinal flowers appeared and told Hazrat Sulaymān their healing properties. And he was the first to have this knowledge, which is of divine origin.

The absolute of the essence of Allah is called *dhāt*. We express this unfathomable absolute with the pronoun *Hū*. Our human minds are incapable of conceiving of or expressing the full reality of Allah. And in considering the nature of God, we must look to the manifold forms of His creation and know Him by His signs.

Each of the divine attributes has a *dhāt*, which is its totality. For example, *ar-Raḥmān* is the totality of every kind of mercy that exists, has ever existed, and will ever exist, in all forms, whether physical, mental, or spiritual, and whether we know of it or do not. Allah, in His mercy, has bestowed untold forms of this mercy throughout the human, angelic, and animal creation. Yet all these untold numbers of manifestations are still only a small part of the *dhāt*, or totality, of Allah's attribute of *ar-Raḥmān*.

This notion of an absolute essence also applies to the human being in relation to the soul (*rūḥ*). This intimate relationship between absolute essence and manifold forms of that essence is duplicated in all of nature. Each flower, tree, and shrub has its physical form and also its essence. The seed of an oak will not produce a willow. All of the specific characteristics of the flower are contained within the seed, within its essence: the height of the plant, the shape of leaves and flowers, the plant's periods of dormancy, color, fragrance, and even its healing characteristics. We learned of some of these essential attributes when we studied the relationship between foods and health.

Our own human absolute essence, or soul, is extracted at the moment of death. Allah has inspired various of His prophets (peace be upon them all) to discover the methods of extracting the souls (*rūḥ*) from flowers, and this knowledge has been preserved in Sufism.

A prominent example is what is called *rūh-i gulāb*, or soul of the rose. It is considered that the absolute perfected essence of the rose exists within the flower itself, just as the perfected essence or soul of a human exists within the body. These essences of flowers are of inestimable value in correcting imbalances in the human being.

The symbol of Sufism itself is the rose, because this flower is considered to be the Mother of Scents and the Queen of the Garden. The placement of the rare and refined beauty and sweetness of the rose blossoms—at the end of a long, stern stem full of prickly thorns—aptly symbolizes the mystic path to Allah the Almighty.

The 124,000 prophets Allah has sent to the world with His Guidance had different bodies but the same soul. Their message to humanity was the same regardless of the physical form they had, the color of their skin, or the language they spoke.

Allah said that the first thing He created in the universe was the soul of prophecy. He said that He made it from the absolute of His own light, called *nūr*. Allah further stated that if He had not created this soul of prophecy, He woud not have created the universe.

After Allah the Almighty made this magnificent soul, it was of such luminous nature and so burning with light that it began to shed drops of perspiration. And from this sweat of the soul of prophecy, Allah made the soul of the rose. This is the actual origin of the art and science of aromatherapy.

Every prophetic tradition uses flowers and their oils in healing. If we consider the nature of flowers themselves, we realize that they are stimulated into growth and subsist primarily by virtue of their relationship with the light rays from the sun, and by means of the process called photosynthesis give off the components of oxygen and air that we use for breath. Flowers require this nourishment of light, as well as that of the soil and rain.

It is said that people used to follow the Prophet Muhammad (s.a.w.s.) and collect the drops of his perspiration, finding them to be the very sweetest smell and fragrance of all, superior to any flower's scent. The reason these droplets were of such elegance is that they contained the essence of his soul.

That magical moment of interconnection between life and nonlife—the moment of birth—is when the soul is activated within the body. Our life span is measured between the first breath and the last breath. At the moment of that first breath, one can find the model for all scents, coming from the skin and breath of infants just after they are born.

The scent of an infant creates the deepest and most profound love and affection in the heart and mind and soul of the person who receives it. There is no one who does not appreciate the intimate fragrance of a newborn. It is an irreplaceably unique smell, and one simply cannot get enough of it. It is of an absolute clarity and purity, and it somehow embodies all of the feelings of helpless trust and reliance upon one superior to the infant, which encapsulates our whole relationship with the Creator, exalted is He.

Babies are born pure and sinless, having within them the divine light and peace; the very essence of the soul of prophecy is within them. No doubt, as they grow into consciousness of the world, they lose their innocence, and the scent dwindles and disappears as they become immersed in the life of the world—in the *maqām an-nafs*.

So it must be remembered when we talk about the essence of flowers that they are imitating the superior scents of the soul of prophecy, from which they are derived.

The soul of a flower may be extracted in several ways: by pressing the oils out of the petals; by distilling water through the petals; or by bonding the oil to a base oil. In all cases, the essence of the flower is drawn out by this process. The word for these essences (or oils containing the essences) is "attar" (from Arabic *ᶜiṭr*). In the West, these are called essential oils, fragrances, absolutes, and sometimes perfumes.

The addition of alcohol to the essence of a flower will kill that essence, and so those oils or remedies containing alcohol are unsuitable for Sufi healing purposes.

When applying attars or essential oils, great care must be exercised because they are in such a concentrated form—not only the active physical ingredients, but also the essence is very strong. For this reason, some attars are diluted before use, in a pure base oil such as olive, sandalwood, or sweet almond.

Ideally, one should use the fresh blossoms of the rose (or other flower), and place a few ounces in a small bowl of spring water for several hours at midday. This will extract the essence, and one need not worry about purity or additives. Or one may eat a few of the fresh petals themselves, as this admits of the least alteration of all. But for the sake of convenience and availability, it is sometimes prudent to keep a supply of a high-quality pure oil on hand.

Because the rose is considered to have the most refined essence of all flowers, it is often used to absorb and convey the *baraka* (blessing) of a saint. People who visit the resting places (*dargah*s) of saint's often place the rose petals on the tomb itself, then retrieve them for later use in healing. Since the soul of the saint is living, the rose essence will imbibe the essence of the saint, which can then be consumed and conveyed into any person with uniformly positive results.

Many Sufi *khanagahs* (monasteries) have rose gardens growing nearby. The Sufis also recite various verses of the Qur'an over rose petals, charging them with even greater healing powers (see following chapters).

Sufi Abu Anees Muhammad Barkat Ali (may Allah be pleased with him), at his spiritual retreat in Pakistan, makes his own soul remedies according to the above methods. From a nearby rose garden, he gathers up fresh petals, over which constant prayers and remembrance of Allah are carried out. These same petals are dried out in a special room in which there are more than 250,000 copies of the Holy Qur'an, as well as one of the four oldest Qur'ans in existence, dating from the time of Hazrat ᶜUthmān (r.a.). The room, which is called the Qur'ān Maḥall (House of the Qur'an), vibrates with the divine presence. The petals are laid out and arranged so as to form the shape of the word *Allah*, and various verses are recited over them for some time, thus maturing them for healing. Even one or two petals of the medicines prepared thus have been demonstrated to effect a cure, as it pleases Allah.

Anyone can utilize this method. Take a clean cloth, preferably of forest-green color, and if not that, blue or white, of large enough size to hold the shape of the word (about three feet by four feet). After reciting *Bismi Llāh ir-Raḥmān, ir-Raḥīm* (In the name of Allah, Most Gracious, Most Merciful), spread out the petals to form the word *Allah*, following exactly the sequence shown in the illustration.

After completing the shape of the word *Allah* in the order indicated, recite over it 786 times, *Bismi Llāh ir-Raḥmān, ir-Raḥim*. If you have the time and inclination, this formula can be recited any number of times. After completing this procedure, you may use the petals for healing.

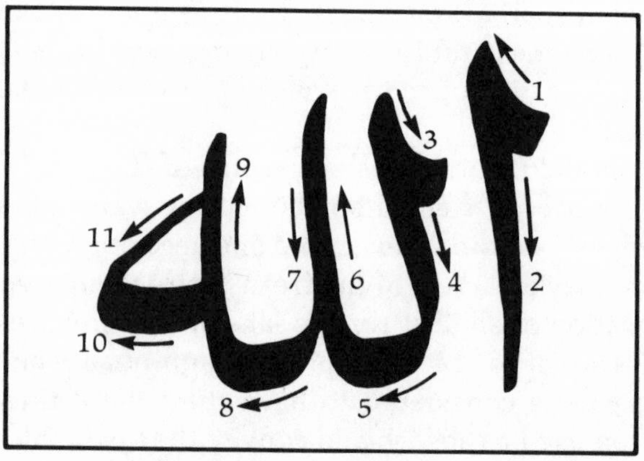

Shape and sequence of writing the word Allāh.

Yā Ḥayyu, yā Qayyūm! Lā ilāha illā anta yā arḥām ar-raḥīmīn! Āmīn! O the Living, O the Everlasting! There is none except You, O the Most Merciful of the Merciful! *Āmīn!*

Although there are perhaps fifty or sixty thousand different plants from which essential oils can be extracted, the Sufis use primarily those which are recommended upon divine information. The attars that will be discussed are amber, frankincense, myrrh, violet, sandalwood, musk, rose, jasmine, hina, ᶜūd, and jannat al-fardaws. All are pure oils except the last, which is a blend.

It is more important to learn to use a few oils very well than not know much at all about hundreds of oils. Even just with these ten oils, there are more than one hundred trillion combinations!

Amber

Oil of amber (*kahrabah* in Persian), or liquid amber, as it is sometimes called, is derived from a species of pine tree (*Picea succinfera*). Many people have had contact with amber stones and beads, and it is this same basic substance that is used in healing. But the stones have hardened for several million more years than the resin, which is used to manufacture the oil.

There are only three locales in the world where authentic amber can be found. Its color varies anywhere from a light, translucent pink to a heavy, dark brown. When we realize that the essential sap of these trees, to become amber, has been preserved for one to six million years, we understand that we are tapping into a very ancient healing energy.

Some people use the sap from trees and distill out the essence. But others, realizing this ancient energy within, prefer to grind down the stones into powder and then heat it to retrieve the essence. This latter form of amber is better for healing, but very, very difficult to locate.

Amber has been fossilized for so long that we even have no way of knowing what other life forms were present. But we do know that the prophets (a.s.) who lived long ago had extraordinary powers of perception and healing. It is said, for example, that one prophet was able to overhear a conversation of ants, at a distance of more than ten miles! It is likely that in addition to being endowed with spiritual powers, they had hidden knowledge of healing plants. Many of these species are now extinct.

Although the best amber comes only from the Near East, Russia, and the Dominican Republic, frequently it is taken to other parts of the world for processing out its essences, for making it into attar. Amber processed in Tunis and the Sudan is remarkably pure, clear, and healing. The Sudanese variety is much hotter than the Tunisian, and thus stronger in effect. It is so thick that it will not pour and must be heated to get it out of the bottle.

A cake amber available from Afghanistan is the best in the world, and not so expensive if purchased in that country. Unfortunately, it is difficult to obtain it at present.

Amber is recommended specifically for any kind of disease or problem associated with the heart. While the rose is considered the Mother of Scents, amber is called the Father (or King) of Scents.

Very little use is made of amber in Western healing today, although it used to be commonly prescribed for heart conditions by medical doctors in the 1920s.

An excellent method of using amber is to put one drop on the tip of the finger and apply it to the point of the "Third Eye" (not in the physical eyes, of course). This is absorbed by the body and stimulates the pineal gland, which activates many of our physiological functions.

Frankincense

The word *incense* comes from the French *encens* and originally meant "frankincense," but it now refers to any kind of fragrant vapor. *Frank* was appended to the word *incens*, to add the meaning of "luxurious" or "expensive." So, to the French, *frankincense* means the very best fragrance.

The original Latin word for incense was *par fumum*, meaning "through smoke." The burning of the oils is a common mode of application, because it further refines the essence, releases it into the air, and makes it easy to disperse over a wide area. It is an effective means of administering scent to the insane, children, or others who cannot or will not participate in smelling the scents.

When an essence is taken in its vaporized form, it travels into the body via the networks of the essences and reaches its goal more easily; whereas if it is swallowed or rubbed on the skin, there are many possibilities that it will not arrive at the desired destination, especially if it goes via the stomach. Digestive juices may annul the healing effects, because alcohol is one of the by-products of normal digestion.

Frankincense is hot in the second degree, but is not quite so hot as amber. It is a little less drying, too.

Frankincense is to this day used in the religious ceremonies of the Catholic Church, and was one of the scents presented to the infant Jesus (a.s.). This is so because frankincense is a very powerful cleanser of the aura and psychic planes.

Myrrh

Myrrh is hot and drying. It was one of the oils commanded by God to Moses (a.s.), and also to Jesus (a.s.), to be one of the ingredients in their healing and holy anointing oil. In ancient times it was used to convey to people a certain internal esoteric teaching, to purify their spiritual environment so that the teachings would have a proper soil in which to be planted.

Myrrh is mentioned in the Qur'an as having specific healing properties. Again, there are several varieties, but that from Tunis and Morocco seems to be of first quality.

Violet

Violet is cold and moist in the first degree, and thus can be considered mild in its action. Violet leaves, flowers, and oils are featured in a great number of healing formulas.

Sandalwood

Sandal is cold and dry in the second degree. The best and most famous oil of sandal comes from Mysore, India. It is used in many conditions, frequently for genital and urinary tract infections. Sandal is also used as the base oil into which other oils are extracted or blended. It is a very good base because it evaporates very slowly and does not spoil over time. In fact, aged sandalwood is better than fresh.

Sandalwood is recommended whenever serious meditation and spiritual practices are being undertaken, because it is quieting to all of the egotisms of the body, especially those relating to sexual energies.

Musk

It was reported in the Hadith that the Prophet Muhammad (s.a.w.s.) was particularly fond of musk oil. True musk oil is derived from the sexual glands of a kind of deer, found only in remote regions of the world. Musk is hot and dry. Some people refuse to use it because they object to using any animal substance, for anything. Musk, however, does have a definite place in medicine, particularly in healing heart and sexual problems.

Rose

Rose is cold and dry in the second degree. There are perhaps three hundred different species of roses used in aromatherapy. The finest is said by some to be the attar of Bulgarian rose, which retails at about $350 per ounce. Few people stock it. Others consider that some of the first-pressing rose oils from India are superior even to the Bulgarian rose. Their price is about $450 per pound in India. It requires almost 60,000 pounds of rose petals to produce one kilogram (2.2 pounds) of first-pressing rose oil.

The Indians reportedly discovered rose oil at the time of the wedding of Shah Jehan, the one who built the Taj Mahal and Shalimar gardens as a testament of his unyielding love for his wife, Noor Jehan. For the wedding day, the emperor had filled the moat surrounding his castle with rose water, over which the wedding guests were to be ferried. As the sun beat down its heat on the rose water, it caused a natural distillation of the oil, which separated off and floated on top of the rose pond. This was skimmed off, and the Indians have excelled at producing rose oil ever since.

The rose is the most superior of all scents in the floral realm. Rose works simultaneously on the physical, emotional, and spiritual bodies, purifying and uplifting all three. It is the least toxic oil. One can make a delicious summer drink by adding one drop of rose oil to a gallon of water. Shake it up, and then take *one drop* of that liquid and add it to another fresh gallon of water. The resulting mixture is highly refreshing. This single drop still carries the power to scent the water, even though it has been diluted almost a million times.

Jasmine

Jasmine is cold and dry. The flowers of jasmine are cold, but the essential oil is heating. This is an important consideration: that not all substances work in the same way in all forms, just as water and ice are chemically the same but quite different in their effects. It is also true that flowers and their oils do not work the same way in humans as they do in animals: what is heating to a human may be cooling to a fish. This fact makes random experiments on animals a questionable practice at best. Jasmine is the scent favored by the shaykhs of the famous whirling mystic dancers of Turkey. Its special quality is its unparalleled ability to uplift the mood and lessen mental depression.

Hina

Hina (pronounced *heena*) is the oil extracted from the flowers of the henna plant. Hina is very difficult to obtain in the United States. It is considered one of the finest and most refined oils in the world, and its price reflects that. In India, a dram of first-quality hina oil (about a teaspoon) costs about $100. This is because it is usually aged over a long time, and improves with aging. I have seen catalogues advertising it for as much as $1,000 a pound. But one can obtain various hina oils that are blended, thus bringing the price into reach of the average person.

The curious thing about hina (and some of the other oils as well) is that the liking for its fragrance is an acquired one: many people on first smelling it find it repulsive.

ᶜŪd

The rare and costly oil known as ᶜūd is taken from the wood of the aloeswood tree. The best ᶜūd comes from India. Its cost can be as high as $800 per dram. However, those familiar with its effects do not find the price a consideration.

It could be stated that ᶜūd is enjoyed only by those of the higher evolutions of the soul; indeed, its application is usually restricted to imbalances of the last three stations.

Jannat al-Fardaws

Although a blend, jannat al-fardaws is very popular among the Sufis. It is said that a Sufi *ᶜaṭṭār*, or perfumer, one day entered the Fardaws—the Highest Heaven—in his mystical exertions. Once there, he experienced a particular fragrance. Upon recovering his normal state of mind, he reproduced this fragrance, thus the name: Gateway to the Highest Heaven.

APPLICATION OF OILS

The most common method of using essential oils among the Sufis is to rub a small amount of oil over the extended right hand, palms down. This is the etiquette of receiving an oil offered by a shaykh. Then the oil is rubbed over the beard or chin, across the front of the shirt, and onto the wrists.

A second method of applying the oil, particularly when a mental or emotional condition is being treated, is the following. Put one or two drops of the oil onto a piece of cotton about the size of the end of a cotton swab stick (do not use the stick, however). Then insert the cotton wad into the ridgelike ledge of the ear, just above the ear opening (*not inside the ear*). The illustration shows the correct placement of the oil. This must be done in the *right* ear, not the left. In the right ear, at this point of placement, five cranial nerves come together to form a nerve mass, or ganglia. This is an important point in other systems of medicine as well, such as Chinese acupuncture, where it is called *shen wen*, one of the important life-regulating points.

Now that we understand something about oils, we can assign the oils to be used in each of the stages of the soul's evolution—the stages of egotism, heart, soul, divine secrets, proximity, and union. Each of the stations, their imbalances, and resulting conditions are given in the next section, with the proper oil to be used for each.

Some readers may wonder why I do not suggest applying the oils internally for physical diseases. Although there is a science of utilizing attars and essential oils in this way, I present here the applications which are intended to affect the emotional and spiritual centers because that is where the disease conditions *originate*. Another book presenting the applications of oils for physical conditions is in preparation.

Generally speaking, the oils may be simply smelled for effect in all of the stations of the soul and their imbalances. However, one will find them also effective when added to massage oils and rubbed over the entire body, in the stations of egotism and the heart. The other stations require simply inhalation of the fragrance.

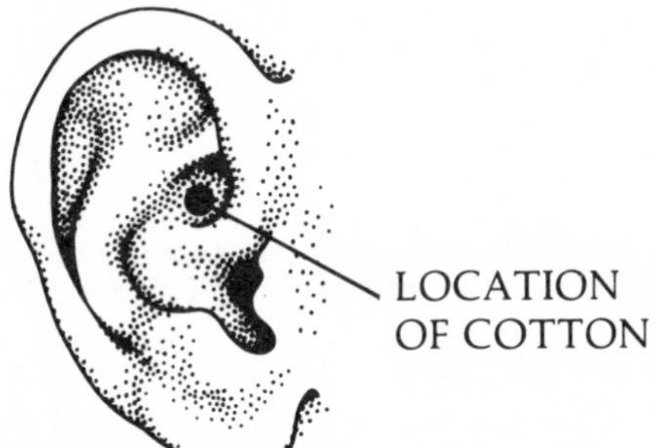

Applying oil drops on cotton to ear.

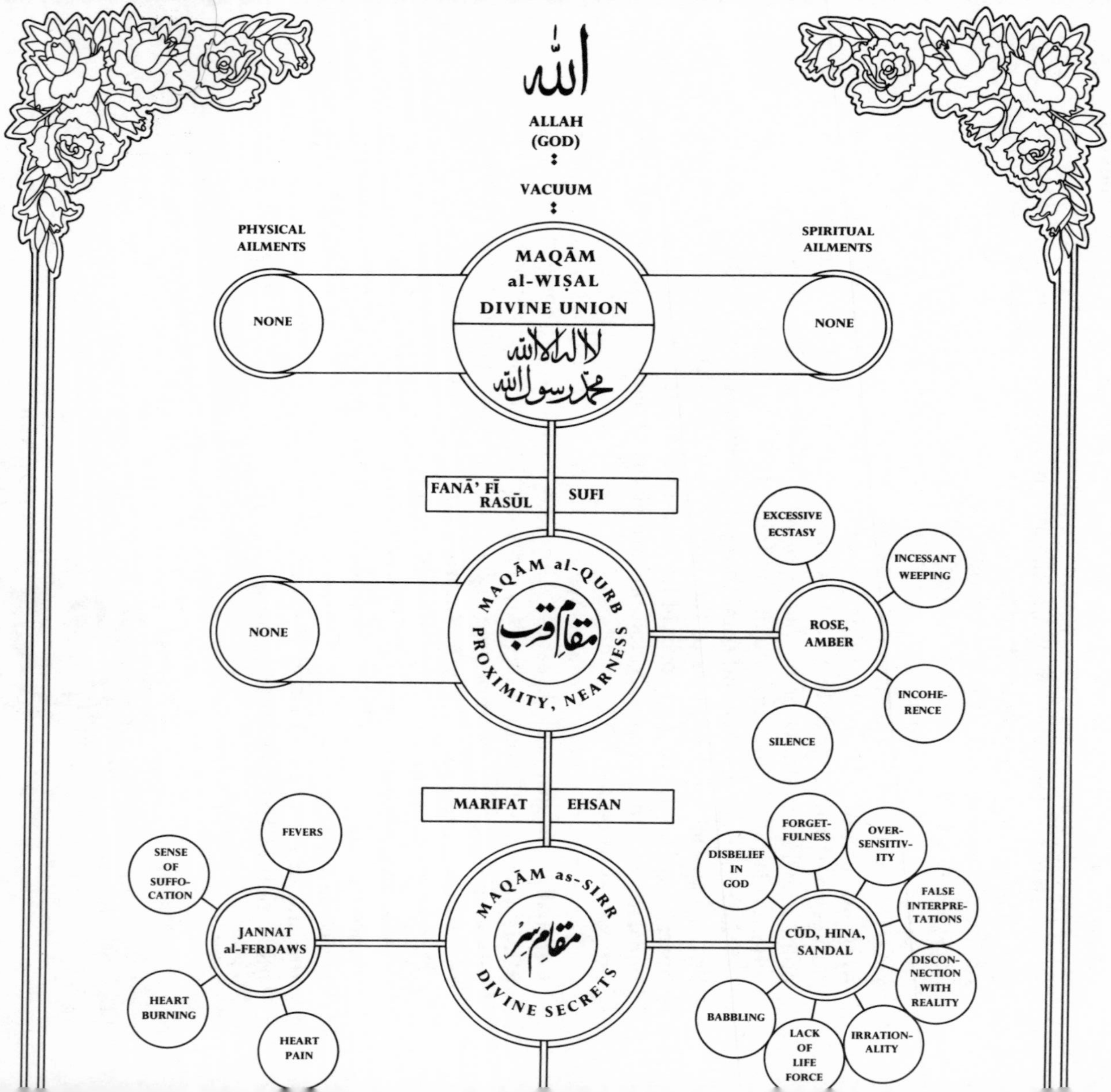

الله
ALLAH
(GOD)
VACUUM
PHYSICAL AILMENTS
SPIRITUAL AILMENTS
MAQĀM al-WIṢAL DIVINE UNION
لا اله الا الله محمد رسول الله
NONE
NONE
FANĀ' FĪ RASŪL
SUFI
MAQĀM al-QURB PROXIMITY, NEARNESS
مقام قرب
NONE
ROSE, AMBER
EXCESSIVE ECSTASY
INCESSANT WEEPING
INCOHE-RENCE
SILENCE
MARIFAT
EHSAN
MAQĀM as-SIRR DIVINE SECRETS
مقام سر
JANNAT al-FERDAWS
FEVERS
SENSE OF SUFFO-CATION
HEART BURNING
HEART PAIN
CŪD, HINA, SANDAL
DISBELIEF IN GOD
FORGET-FULNESS
OVER-SENSITIV-ITY
FALSE INTERPRE-TATIONS
DISCON-NECTION WITH REALITY
IRRATION-ALITY
LACK OF LIFE FORCE
BABBLING

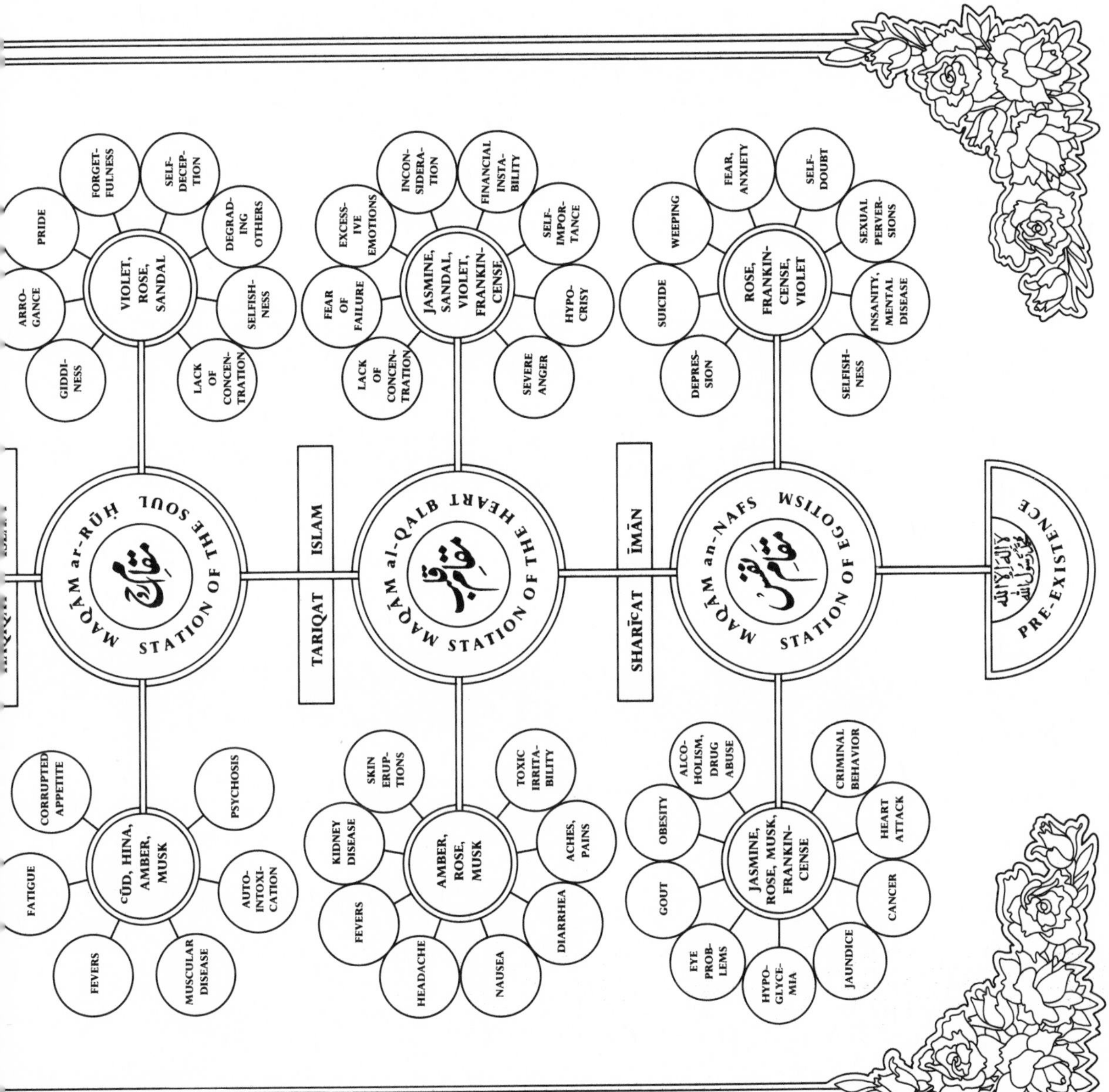

MAQĀM ar-RŪH — STATION OF THE SOUL

- ARROGANCE
- PRIDE
- FORGETFULNESS
- SELF-DECEPTION
- DEGRADING OTHERS
- SELFISHNESS
- LACK OF CONCENTRATION
- GIDDINESS
- VIOLET, ROSE, SANDAL

- FATIGUE
- CORRUPTED APPETITE
- PSYCHOSIS
- AUTO-INTOXICATON
- MUSCULAR DISEASE
- FEVERS
- ‘ŪD, HINA, AMBER, MUSK

TARIQAT — ISLAM

MAQĀM al-QALB — STATION OF THE HEART

- EXCESSIVE EMOTIONS
- INCONSIDERATION
- FINANCIAL INSTABILITY
- SELF-IMPORTANCE
- HYPOCRISY
- SEVERE ANGER
- LACK OF CONCENTRATION
- FEAR OF FAILURE
- JASMINE, SANDAL, VIOLET, FRANKINCENSE

- SKIN ERUPTIONS
- TOXIC IRRITABILITY
- ACHES, PAINS
- DIARRHEA
- NAUSEA
- HEADACHE
- FEVERS
- KIDNEY DISEASE
- AMBER, ROSE, MUSK

SHARĪ‘AT — ĪMĀN

MAQĀM an-NAFS — STATION OF EGOTISM

- WEEPING
- FEAR, ANXIETY
- SELF-DOUBT
- SEXUAL PERVERSIONS
- INSANITY, MENTAL DISEASE
- SELFISHNESS
- DEPRESSION
- SUICIDE
- ROSE, FRANKINCENSE, VIOLET

- ALCOHOLISM, DRUG ABUSE
- CRIMINAL BEHAVIOR
- HEART ATTACK
- CANCER
- JAUNDICE
- HYPOGLYCEMIA
- EYE PROBLEMS
- GOUT
- OBESITY
- JASMINE, ROSE, MUSK, FRANKINCENSE

PRE-EXISTENCE

It should be remembered that the intended result is not to attack a disease, but rather to create an irresistible invitation of kindness and sweetness to the next stage of evolution.

The final thing to remember is that when working with emotions and spiritual actions, the results are in accord with nature; that is, they work in conformity with the body's own healing energies, and not abruptly. As a great Sufi once said, "Patience is the key to joy."

11

The Universe of the Breath

And remember when thy Lord said unto
the angels:
Lo! I am creating a mortal
out of potter's clay of black mud altered.
So, when I have made him
and have breathed into him of My
spirit . . .

Qur'an 15:28–29

The Qur'anic verse above reveals in a very condensed form the entire mystic relationship between God and His human creation. He says that He made the human being out of the elements and then breathed life into the body. The Qur'anic words used here are significant.

Allah uses the word *nafas* for His own breath, and He uses the word *rūḥ* for His own soul. These same words are used to mean the human breath and human soul—confirming the fact that we are originally from Allah, of Allah, for Allah, and in the end will return to Allah.

Of all of the physical realities that have a bearing upon health, that which is least often considered in medicine and healing is the breath. The breath has the following important relations with health:

1. It is the agent upon which the divine permission (*idhn*) is borne.
2. Breath is responsible for conveying the divine attributes from the heart to the various centers of the mind, body, and soul.
3. Breath creates the equilibrium and harmony of the temperaments of the body.
4. Breath carries life-supporting elements from the exterior of the body to the interior physiological functions.

Breath is not synonymous with air, nor with oxygen. Breath is that which emerges from the divine origin and has as its essence the temperament of the celestial realms. Breath is a luminous substance, a ray of light; breath is the life force of God Himself!

Breath is the regulator of joy, sadness, delight, anger, jealousy, and other emotions. Both the quantity and quality of breath have a definite and direct effect upon human health. This is so because various physical events can alter or in a sense cover over the divine essence that is being conveyed on the breath. Industrial pollutants, alcoholic beverages, and various foods can all intermingle with the breath and disturb its intended purity of action.

All of these actions are changed by age, climate, and habits. An example will make this clear. When one experiences great depression, there is a weakening of the natural powers and a concentration of the breath. This concentration causes a violent aggregation of the breath, which consequently obliterates part of the natural heat and gives rise to an imbalance of coldness. Depending upon how prolonged the depression is, the cold imbalance can extend into one or many organs of the body, thus producing varying degrees of disease.

The emotions of dread and the effects associated with great and impending danger also dissipate the natural heat. Anger will cause an increase in the amount of yellow bile essence created. If the anger is sustained, the diseases associated with excess yellow bile will occur.

Therefore, medicines must be chosen for their effect on the breath and its temperament (or its altered temperament). This is why compound medicines are frequently used, to balance not only the physical symptoms but also the underlying temperaments of the physiological essences *and* the essences of the breath.

This is also why flower essences, in the form of attars, are so effective in producing cures. It is vital that they be given at the same time as medicines that strictly affect the physical symptoms. Flowers have the greatest capacity to rebalance the breath and the internal essential temperaments.

The breath is the nexus between our Creator and ourselves. The healing methods of the Sufis have placed more importance upon the breath than on any other factor of life.

In February 1979, I received a letter from my old friend Yunus Maharaj, the head of the families who attend to the *dargah* of our Chishti headquarters at Ajmer. "Man does not come to earth to stay forever," he wrote. My heart was pounding, knowing what was to follow. "Hazrat Maulana Sufi Darveesh Wahiduddin Begg completed his breathing practices on the 12th of Rabī^{c}a^{c} al-Awwal, A.H. 1400. It was an auspicious time, just after sunset. The day was more auspicious still: it was the birthday of the Prophet (s.a.w.s.)." Although there were many feelings I experienced in association with the passing of my shaykh (may Allah cover him with mercy), I was struck by the unique view Yunus Maharaj had expressed to me: that life, considered from its beginning to end, is one continuous set of breathing practices. This is the view of the Sufis.

The Holy Qur'an, in addition to all else that it may be, is a set of breathing practices. In fact, the very first command of Almighty God was to recite the Qur'an. The first verses that were revealed by Gabriel to Prophet Muhammad (s.a.w.s.) were as follows:

Iqra' bismi Rabbik alladhī khalaq
Khalaqal insāna min ᶜalaq
Iqra' wa Rabbukal-Akram
Alladhī 'allama bil-qalam
'Allamal insana mā lam yaᶜlam.

Recite! In the name of Thy Lord
Who createth man from a drop of sensitized blood
Recite! And thy Lord is Most Bounteous,
Who teacheth by the pen
Teacheth man that which he knew not.

The Arabic word *iqra'* is rendered here as "recite" because it means to read from some book, from actual letters. Now, the Prophet (s.a.w.s.) was an *ummī*, an unlettered one who could not read or write, so the command seemed puzzling, even terrifying, to him at the time. But the Holy Prophet (s.a.w.s.) was able to memorize each of the verses as it came to him, and thus could "read" it from his memory, although actual physical written copies were produced during the lifetime of Muhammad (s.a.w.s.).

One of the Companions of the Prophet related this comment by Muhammad (s.a.w.s.) on the value of reciting the Qur'an: "Reciting the Qur'an out of memory carries one thousand degrees of religious merit, while reading the Qur'an from the Book itself increases [the merit] up to two thousand degrees."

The benefits and effects of reading the Qur'an are like a seed that eventually sends out twigs, branches, roots, and leaves of sustenance in every direction. The Hadith state: "Whoever reads the Qur'an and acts upon what is contained in it, his parents will be made to wear a crown on the Day of Judgment, the brilliance of which will exceed that of the sun, if it were brought down into your houses." So, if that is the reward for the parents, what do you think is the reward for the person who acts upon it himself?

The most important consideration regarding the Qur'an is that Allah states in the Book that it is not of human origin; it consists of the actual pre-eternal, uncreated speech of Allah Himself. As such, no other book exists which carries the degree of perfection and balance in its words. Even the most disinterested observer cannot fail to be impressed upon hearing the Qur'an recited. It is of surpassing beauty, melody, and majesty.

Another important point about the Qur'an is that within the first seven lines, virtually all of the sounds that occur in Arabic are uttered. One of these letters is *ghayn*, which when uttered causes a kind of growling, guttural sound in the back of the throat. Each letter sets off a vibratory pattern that travels in a specific direction, lasts a specific duration, and produces specific physical, mental, and spiritual effects. The sound of the letter *ghayn* (and also *khā'*, *ᶜayn*, and others) is usually not made in the English language. This means that the effects associated with such letters are not felt unless one recites the Arabic. It is a bit curious that most of the sounds that occur in Arabic and not in English are associated with the sounds of choking in English!

Even more important, the various combinations of vowels and consonants combine to stimulate and disperse the divine attributes throughout the body of the reciter in perfect measure. One of the attributes is *al-Ghafūr* (the Forgiver), which contains the letter *ghayn*. One who never recites this letter is deprived of the full measure of forgiveness in his or her own soul.

There are three basic vowel sounds in Arabic: the letters *alif, waw,* and *yā'*.

Name of Vowel Sound	Pronunciation	Symbol
Alif	ā as in *father*	ا
Yā'	ī as in *machine*	و
Waw	ū as in *you*	ي

All languages utilize these three basic long vowel sounds, and they can be thought of as universal harmonic constants, uttered not only by humans, but by every being in Creation. Once one has become attuned to these sounds, one can listen in on the conversations of all of nature!

The vibrations of these three sounds have different effects. The long vowel sound of *ā* travels downward and stimulates the heart, the repository of divine attributes. The long *ī* travels upward and stimulates the pineal gland, which is not fully understood by Western science, but is felt to be responsible for activation of the life forces. And the long sound of *ū* resonates on the outer rim of the pursed lips, and intermingles with the *idhn* of Allah, as His permission for our lives unites with our inhaled and exhaled breaths.

These sounds are not particularly sung or spoken, but are expressed in a special recitation, which is achieved correctly after some time of reading from the Qur'an. In time, these sounds resonate their essence in the tone box of the soul. This may seem a vague manner of expressing such things, but until and unless one experiences it, such descriptions must suffice.

In addition to the foregoing considerations of sound and breath, the Qur'an contains yet another unique feature that transforms it into a full set of breathing practices.

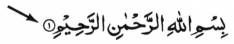

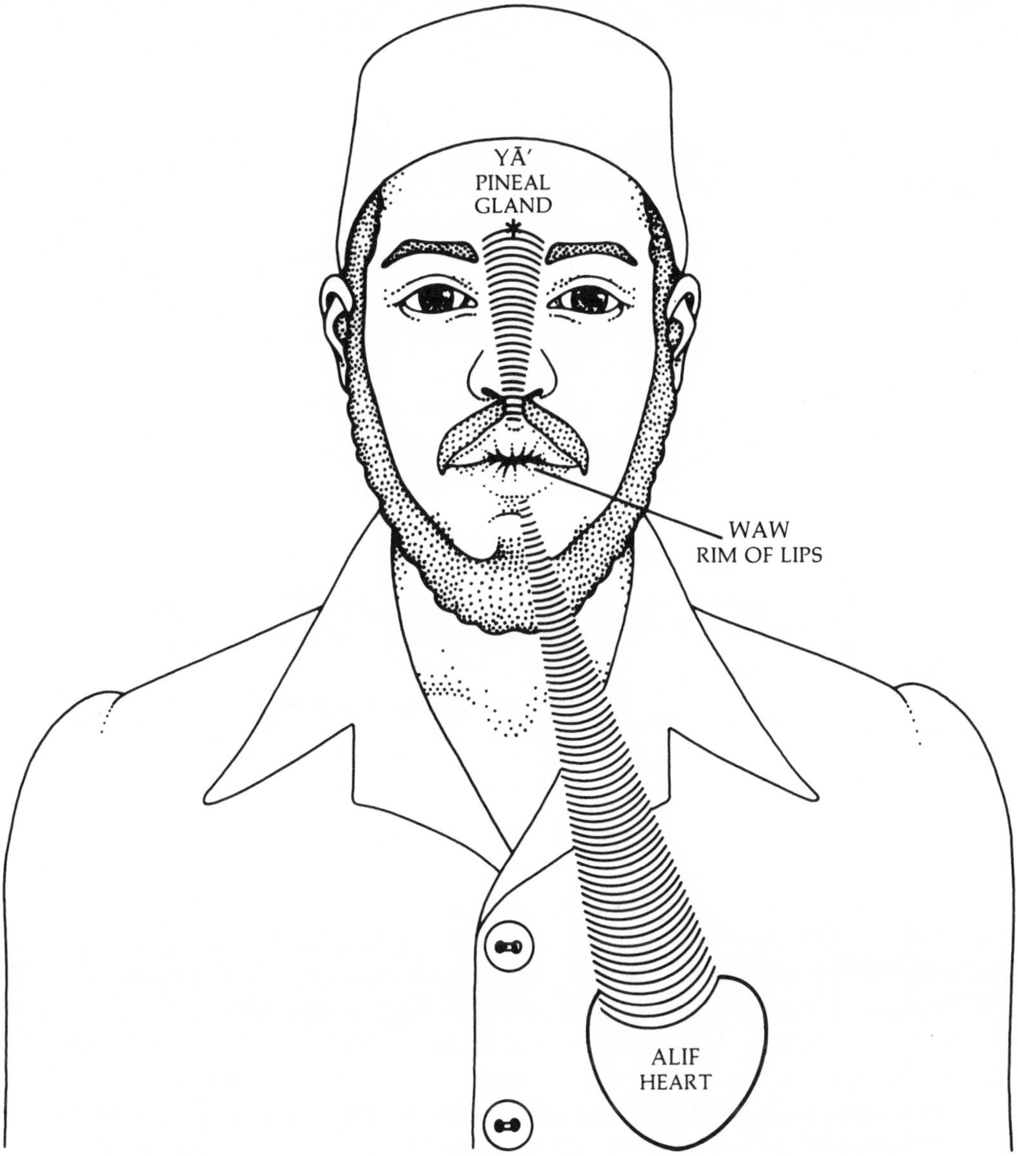

The illustration above shows the point of origin and direction of travel of the vibratory tones associated with each vowel sound.

Appearing as punctuation marks in most editions of the Holy Qur'an (although not in editions for native Arabic speakers, who already know them) are various marks in the text. One set of these markings is called *waqf*, which means "pause" and indicates where the reciter must stop and take a full breath. The main *waqf* mark is a small circle, as shown by an arrow in the following line:

→ بِسْمِ اللّٰهِ الرَّحْمٰنِ الرَّحِيْمِ ①

المنزل ١

بِسْمِ اللّٰهِ الرَّحْمٰنِ الرَّحِيْمِ ۝١

اَلْحَمْدُ لِلّٰهِ رَبِّ الْعٰلَمِيْنَ ۝٢ لا

الرَّحْمٰنِ الرَّحِيْمِ ۝٣ لا

مٰلِكِ يَوْمِ الدِّيْنِ ۝٤ ط

اِيَّاكَ نَعْبُدُ وَاِيَّاكَ نَسْتَعِيْنُ ۝٥ ط

اِهْدِنَا الصِّرَاطَ الْمُسْتَقِيْمَ ۝٦ لا

صِرَاطَ الَّذِيْنَ اَنْعَمْتَ عَلَيْهِمْ ۙ غَيْرِ الْمَغْضُوْبِ

ع عَلَيْهِمْ وَلَا الضَّآلِّيْنَ ۝٧ ع

Main Waqf *Marks in Sūrat al-Fātiḥah*

As an example, in Sūrat al-Fātiḥah, which opens the Qur'an, there are seven of these marks, placed after each of the seven *ayats*, or verses. One who is reciting at the elementary stages *must* stop whenever coming to this mark. This pause forces each line to be of a specified length, which is the same length as it appeared in the original form revealed to the Prophet Muhammad (s.a.w.s.).

However, realizing that some persons have greater capacity than others, Allah has allowed several forms of recitation of the Qur'an, each appropriate to a different capacity for breath and spiritual evolution. Thus, additional marks occur, allowing several of the *ayats* to be recited without the main pauses. Thus, the length of time of recitation may be as short as a few seconds or as long as two minutes.

The correct seven main breath pauses for the opening *sūrah* are reproduced in the accompanying illustration. Anyone who is learning the Qur'an does so by initially following these main breath pauses.

The signs inside the circles indicate the number of the *ayat*. The marks above the circles designate which of the stops are compulsory to obey and which can be gone past. The sign of *lam-alif* (لا) means that to stop is necessary, although it can be optional. When encountering this sign, one may continue on past all *lam-alifs*, until one arrives at the sign of *ṭā* (ط), which marks the compulsory stop for the second level of reciting. Another mode of reciting allows reciting past the *ṭā* as well, stopping only when the sign of *ʿayn* (ع) appears over the circle. Thus, one may recite the entire Sūrat al-Fātiḥah using seven breaths, three breaths, or one breath. In some of the *ayat*s, these breath pauses allow for recitations lasting almost two full minutes. It is indeed astonishing to hear the Qur'an recited in this manner.

Furthermore, there are additional levels of recitation which involve prolonging the breaths and focus upon certain vowels and consonants. One would of necessity require years to attain complete mastery of the modes of reciting the Holy Qur'an. Persons attaining this mastery are called *qāri'*, and have committed the entire Qur'an to memory by this stage.

For the Sufi aspirant, the first requirement is knowledge of the correct modes of reciting the verses of the Holy Qur'an. The ascensions of ecstasy produced thereby can only be imagined. There are more than a few reports of shaykhs expiring while engaged in listening to a recitation of, or themselves reciting, the Holy Qur'an. Shaykh Bayazid Bisṭamī (r.a.) once noted that it was the greatest mystery to him that the person who recited the call to prayer did not die from it.

Obviously, not every person, particularly a novice, can achieve full recitation of the Qur'an within a short time. In order to accelerate the effects of the Qur'an—in its effects upon body, mind, and soul—the Sufis resort to use of the divine names, which condense and compress the effects of longer recitations into a brief space.

It is here that we step off into the realm of the divine realities, where only true and great faith will sustain one.

12

Ta^{c}wīdh: The Merciful Prescriptions

We send down stage by stage in the Qur'an that which is a healing and a mercy to those who believe. . . .

Qur'an 17:82

The Sufis use four things in their treatment of diseases: prayers, medicines, practicing certain things, and giving certain things up.

The practicing and giving up of certain things derive from the primary religious injunctions of the Holy Qur'an. They include abstaining from pork and alcohol, performing daily prayers, cleansing the body by ablutions, and many other things. The use of medicines (including foods and herbs) has been noted as acceptable, and even encouraged, by the Prophet Muhammad (s.a.w.s.). Although all of these actions are necessary, even compulsory, for health, the Sufis consider prayer to be the most superior kind of medicine.

In addition to the various prayers that the Sufis perform daily, they have knowledge of specific verses of the Qur'an, and the names of various attributes of God, which are combined in particular ways to effect cures. This form of healing is called the science of *ta^{c}wīdh*. The word is derived from the verb *^{c}ādha*, "to flee to God for refuge."

The science of *ta^{c}wīdh* combines all the aspects of prayer, breath, and sound. The procedures involved in making these formulations may become complex. The reason these formulas work will be taken up in Chapter 14, "The Origin of Miracles." But the actual mechanics of making *ta^{c}wīdh* can be demonstrated to some extent.

In the writing and utilizing of the sacred *ta^{c}wīdh*, numbers often form a central part of the finished *ta^{c}wīdh*. To the casual observer, these numbers seem somewhat incomprehensible, without any sequential or other significance.

NUMERICAL VALUES FOR ARABIC ALPHABET

Letter (Basic Form)	Numerical Value	Name and Transcription	Letter (Basic Form)	Numerical Value	Name and Transcription
ا	1	*alif*	ض	800	*ḍāḍ: ḍ*
ب	2	*bā: b*	ط	9	*ṭā: ṭ*
ت	400	*tā: t*	ظ	900	*ẓā: ẓ*
ث	500	*thā: th*	ع	70	*ᶜayn: ᶜ*
ج	3	*jīm: j*	غ	1,000	*ghayn: gh*
ح	8	*ḥā: ḥ*	ف	80	*fā: f*
خ	600	*khā: kh*	ق	100	*qāf: q*
د	4	*dāl: d*	ك	20	*kāf: k*
ذ	700	*dhāl: dh*	ل	30	*lām: l*
ر	200	*rā: r*	م	40	*mīm: m*
ز	7	*zā': z*	ن	50	*nūn: n*
س	60	*sīn: s*	ه	5	*hā: h*
ش	300	*shīn: sh*	و	6	*waw: w*
ص	90	*ṣād: ṣ*	ي	10	*yā': y*

Affiliated with the Arabic alphabet is an elaborate system of numerology through which each letter is assigned a numerical value, thus making possible the expression of any written statement by a corresponding number or set of numbers. This science is called *abjad*. The use of numbers has several practical reasons. Often the verse of the Qur'an intended for use may be so long as to preclude its being written out entirely in longhand. Second, there may not be time to write it out, if a formulation is needed within minutes rather than hours or days. A third reason is that, although the Sufis disseminate their healing missions among all humankind without distinctions of any kind, the actual text or letters of the Qur'an have a special sanctity and deserve special forms of care and respect. This being the case, one who does not know the special modes of respecting the Qur'an should not be allowed contact with it. In such cases, numbers can be substituted for the actual verses of the Qur'an without concern for the possibility of loss of or damage to the divine verses.

Thus, the Qur'anic verse *Bismi Llāh ir-Raḥmān, ir-Raḥīm* may be expressed as the number 786. The name Allah is represented by the number 66. The assignation of values to each letter is according to the accompanying table.

There are several ways in which these letters may be represented in transliteration, depending on the original language, whether Arabic, Turkish, Persian, or whatever. The number values are the same, regardless of the symbols used for transliteration.

Applying the values for each individual letter above, we can now compute the number of Allah as 66 by the method illustrated on the following page.

It should be noted that some vowel sounds (*fatḥah*, *kaṣrah*, *ḍammah*) are not written in Arabic script, but are sounded when recited. These vowel sounds are not computed in the numerical values.

In the realm of healing, some of the full Qur'anic verses are written out in number form, as are some of the divine attributes. For example, Sūrat al-Fātiḥah is represented by the numerical chart below:

2340	2343	2346	2332
2345	2343	2339	2344
2344	2348	2341	2338
2342	2337	2335	2347

Clearly understand that it is not the piece of paper or numbers or symbols that do any healing. Such a concept is as erroneous as it is dangerous, for it undermines the exclusiveness of God. It is Allah the Almighty alone who has conceived, designed, and made these formulations available, and it is by His Permission alone that they have effect in human affairs.

الله

Allāh = alif + lam + lam + ha +
1 + 30 + 30 + 5 = 66

The number for *Bismi Llāh ir-Raḥmān, ir-Raḥīm* is computed as follows:

The totals:

40	60	2
م	س	ب
MĪM	*SĪN*	*BĀ*

Bism: 2 + 60 + 40 = 102

5	30	30	1
ه	ل	ل	ا
HĀ	*LĀM*	*LĀM*	*ALIF*

Allāh: 1 + 30 + 30 + 5 = 66

50	40	8	200	30	1
ن	م	ح	ر	ل	ا
NŪN	*MĪM*	*ḤĀ*	*RĀ*	*LĀM*	*ALIF*

ir-Raḥmān: 1 + 30 + 200 + 8 + 40 + 50 = 329

40	10	8	200	30	1
م	ي	ح	ر	ل	ا
MĪM	*YĀ'*	*ḤĀ*	*RĀ*	*LĀM*	*ALIF*

ir-Raḥīm: 1 + 30 + 200 + 8 + 10 + 40 = 289

Total = 786

The formulations are constructed in several ways: they may be written on a piece of paper, voiced as a silent prayer, spoken aloud as a prayer, written on glass and the ink washed off and drunk as medicine, affixed to some part of the body, or buried in the ground, among other methods. Sometimes they are recited within the shaykh and dispersed on his breath, whence, upon arriving as a vibratory pattern on the breath of the patient, they have their effect.

As many as several thousand of these formulas are in use, and one must receive special training in the methods of writing and preparing them correctly. This special training would include, besides knowledge of Arabic, a solid grounding in the external teachings of the Holy Qur'an, the identities of the angelic servants whose duties are particular to healing, the proper times of prayer, and, of course, an ability to correctly diagnose the root cause of the disease on the spiritual realm so that the remedy will have its desired effect.

Not all shaykhs possess the same knowledge. Some specialize in one or several disease conditions, such as jaundice, blindness, insanity, or others. A patient may go to one shaykh for guidance and then be referred by him to another shaykh, one who has the requisite formulas to heal the person.

The shaykh writing out *ta^{c}wīdh* must be very pious, devoid of materialistic intent. The writer must also be maintained in the state of purity, or *wuḍū*. The formulas are written in India ink, and sometimes with vegetable inks of red or green color. Once the *ta^{c}wīdh* is prepared, it is placed inside a metal, cloth, or leather container and worn on some part of the body. Some of the *ta^{c}wīdh* are for a limited time, while others are worn for years. Once their effect is achieved, they must be buried in a safe place.

Because many physical diseases have their origin in emotional imbalances or conditions affecting life-style, the *ta^{c}wīdh* cover a very wide range of applications. For example, if a man is sick because of worry over debts, the healer would provide the patient with a *ta^{c}wīdh* that would increase livelihood, which is the cause of the disease, in the end. *Ta^{c}wīdh* also exist for improving crop output and honey production of bees, to avert calamities, to annul the plots of enemies, for virtually any disease, and for satisfaction in interpersonal relationships.

The following pages reproduce some authentic *ta^{c}wīdh* formulas from the Naqshbandiyyah and Chishtiyyah Sufis in Afghanistan. (It is not permitted to reveal all of the existing *ta^{c}wīdh* or to make the effects available to the general people, lest someone misuse them.)

TA^cWĪDH: The Merciful Prescriptions

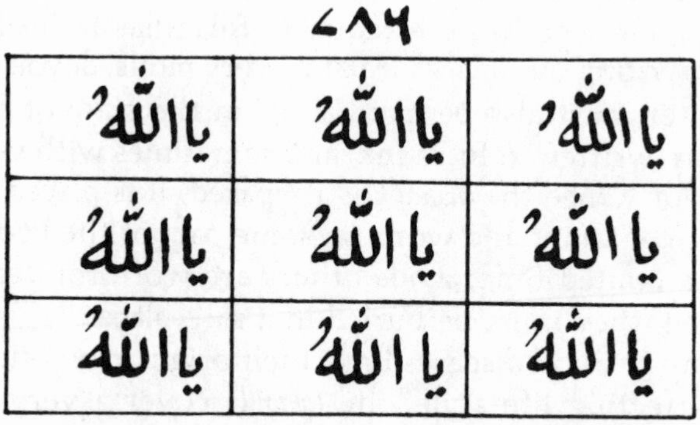

For headache affecting entire head. Worn around neck.

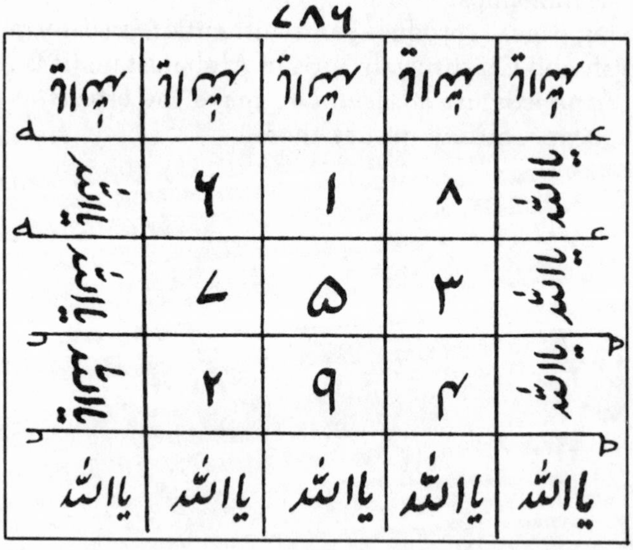

For babies with measles. Worn on throat.

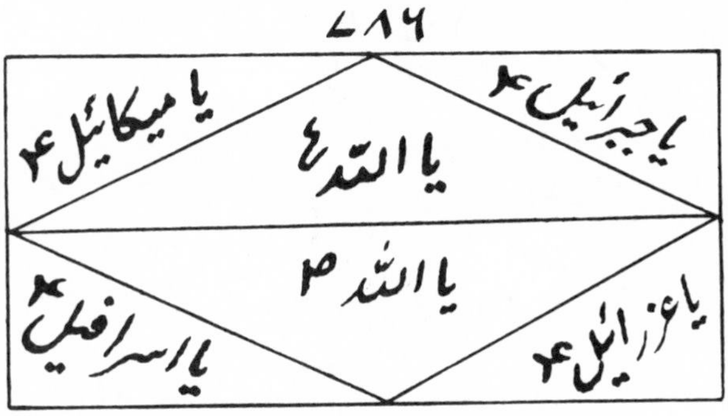

For eye pain. Placed over affected eye.

یاهو	یاهو	یاهو	یاهو
یاهو	یاهو	یاهو	یاهو
یاهو	یاهو	یاهو	یاهو
یاهو	یاهو	یاهو	یاهو

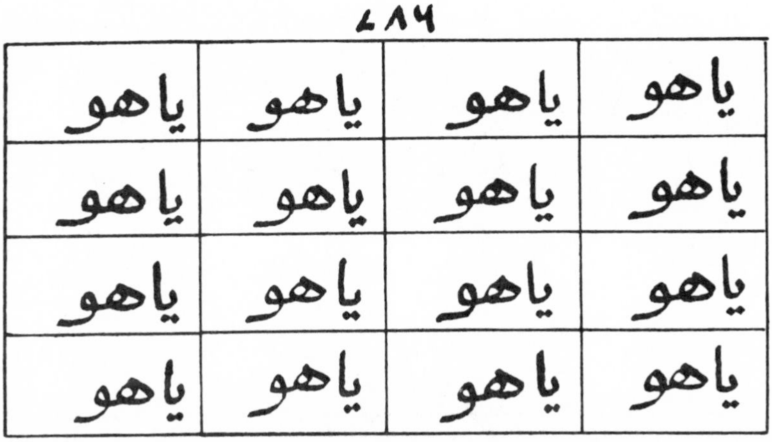

For evil eye or jinns. Worn on the outer clothing.

٥ه٥	٥ه٥	٥ه٥	٥ه٥	٥ه٥	٥ه٥	٥ه٥
٥ه٥	٥ه٥	٥ه٥	٥ه٥	٥ه٥	٥ه٥	٥ه٥
٥ه٥	٥ه٥	٥ه٥	٥ه٥	٥ه٥	٥ه٥	٥ه٥
٥ه٥	٥ه٥	٥ه٥	٥ه٥	٥ه٥	٥ه٥	٥ه٥
٥ه٥	٥ه٥	٥ه٥	٥ه٥	٥ه٥	٥ه٥	٥ه٥

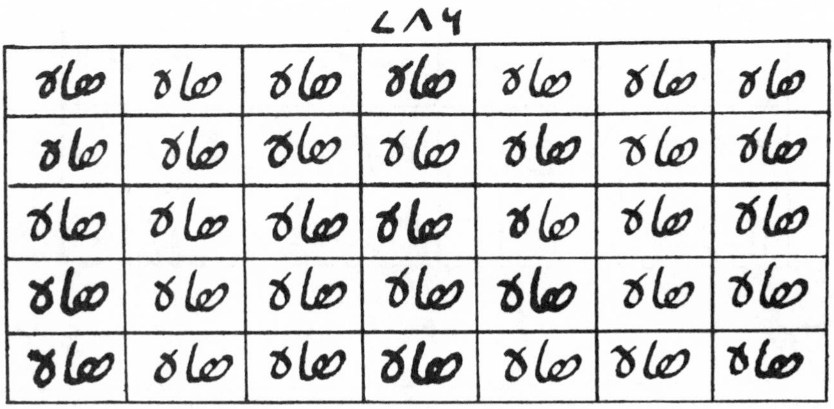

For women who cannot conceive. Written in vegetable ink, washed off, and drunk.

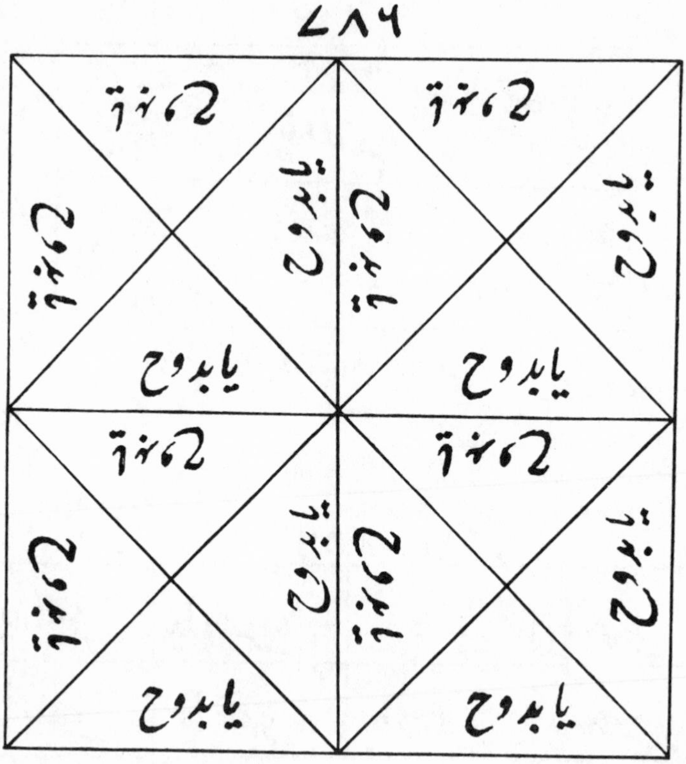

For inflamed eyes. Written on a sunny day. Worn around throat.

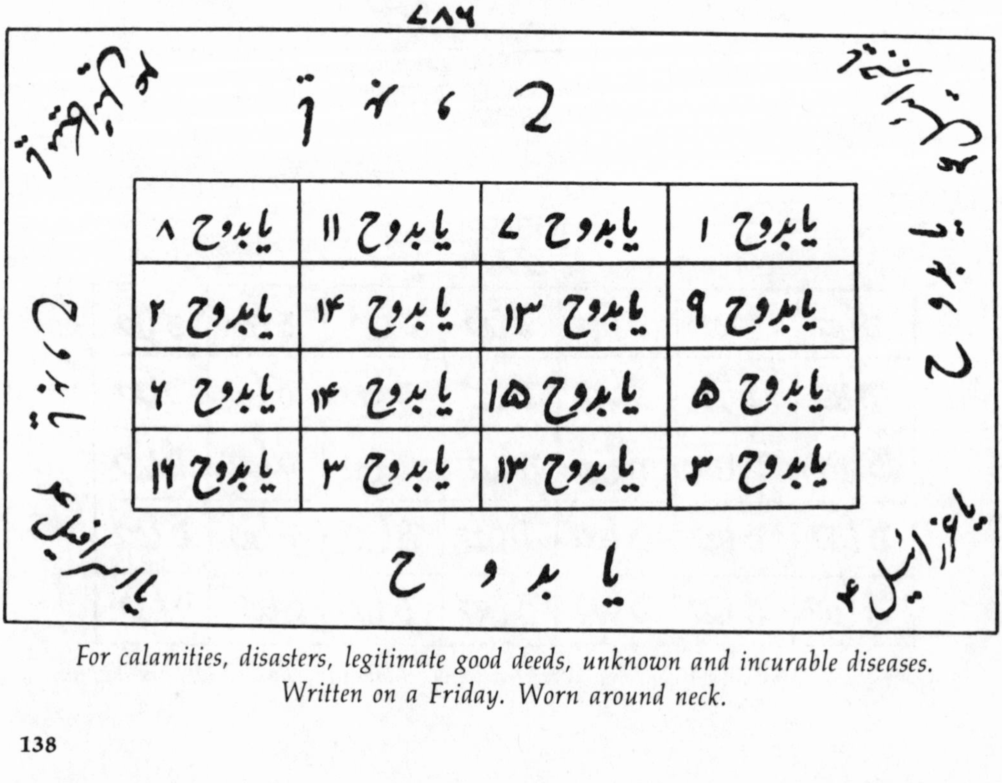

For calamities, disasters, legitimate good deeds, unknown and incurable diseases. Written on a Friday. Worn around neck.

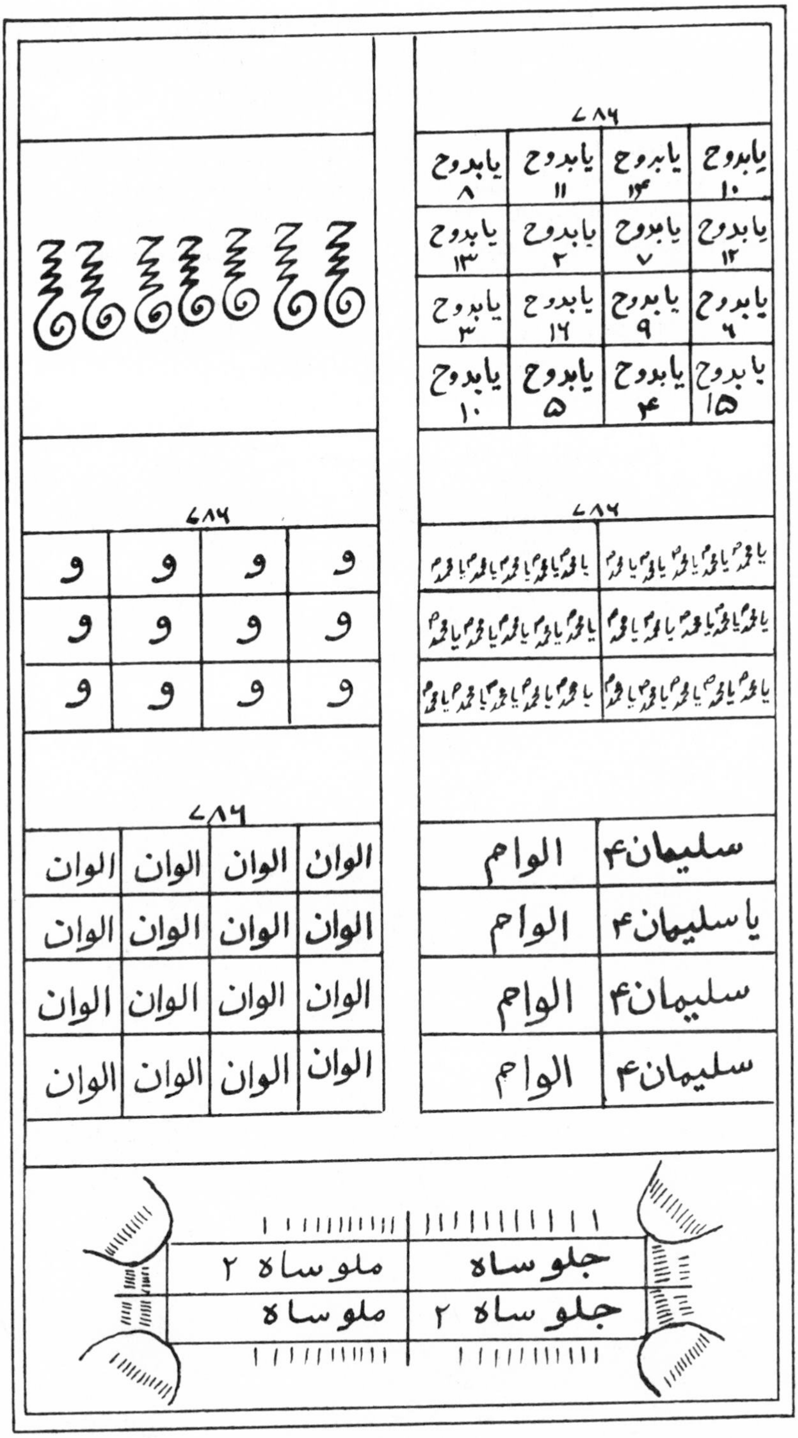

A page from a book of ta^cwīdh illustrating seven different ta^cwīdh for physical diseases.

Let us now turn to the most concentrated and condensed healing formula that exists, the Divine Remembrance, the Celestial Conversation, the Favorite of Allah and the lifeblood and life breath of the Sufis: *dhikr*.

Al-ḥamdu li-Llāh illadhī tawāḍ[c]a kullu shay'in li-[c]azmatihi.
Wal-ḥamdu li-Llāh illadhī dhalla kullu shay'in li-[c]izzatihi.
Wal-ḥamdu li-Llāh illadhī khada[c]a kullu shay'in li-milkihi.
Wal-ḥamdu li-Llāh illadhī astaslama kullu shay'in li-qudratih.

All praise is due to Allah,
before Whose grandeur everything is humbled.
All praise is due to Allah,
before Whose greatness everything is subdued.
All praise is due to Allah,
before Whose dominion everything is abased.
All praise is due to Allah,
before Whose strength
everything surrenders.

13

Dhikr: Divine Remembrance

And men who remember Allah much
and women who remember Allah much,
Allah hath prepared for them forgiveness
and a vast reward.

Qur'an 33:35

The intimate relationship between the Sufi and Allah is contained in the memorable verse from the Qur'an: "If you remember Me, I will remember you" (2:152).

This form of mutual attraction and devotion bespeaks an ulterior form of love which says, in effect, I will relinquish every aspect of my own self and devote myself wholeheartedly and absolutely exclusively to Your pleasure. At any rate, this is the condition in which the Sufi finds himself.

The word used to mean this exclusive and intimate dwelling upon, is *dhikr* (sometimes transliterated as *zikr*). Allah has frequently used this term when revealing the superior forms of worship:

> Remember thy Lord much, and praise Him in the early hours of the night and morning. (3:41)
>
> After you have performed the act of worship [*ṣalāt*], remember Allah standing, sitting, and lying down. (4:103)
>
> Lo! Even I am Allah. There is no god except Me. So serve Me and establish worship for My remembrance. (20:14)
>
> But verily, remembrance of Allah is more important. (29:45)
>
> O ye who believe! Remember Allah with much remembrance. (37:75)

There are dozens more verses in the Holy Qur'an that contain similar testaments to the exalted position in which Allah holds the *dhikr*.

Of course, remembrance in one sense simply could mean any kind of formal thought process alighting upon Allah or His attributes. However, men and women of piety approached the Prophet Muhammad (s.a.w.s.) after these verses were descended and asked for a clarification of the term *dhikr*.

It is reported in the pure Hadith that the Prophet (s.a.w.s.) said: "*Lā ilāha illā Llāhu* is the most excellent of all forms of remembrance of Allah the Almighty." He is also reported to have said that the end of the world will not arrive so long as there is one person left alive reciting *La ilāha illā Llāhu*.

One of the great shaykhs has said: "The ecstasy produced in the heart of the dervishes in their *dhikr* is a kind of turbulence, which is the cause of the waves foaming and breaking upon the shore."

The prophet Moses (a.s.) was told by Allah that *dhikr* is the most preferred of special prayers. Because of its ability to inculcate deep sincerity in the heart of a believer, *Lā ilāha illā Llāhu* is also termed the Purification of Souls.

This sacred formula is also called the Key to Paradise, because the Prophet Muhammad (s.a.w.s.) stated in one of his sermons that the gates of heaven would open for anyone who recited it even once in a lifetime with true sincerity. The word "gates" in the plural was used because there are many gates in heaven, and this formula is the key to all of them.

In short, there is nothing greater in the sight of Allah than this remembrance of Him, exalted is He: *Lā ilāha illā Llāhu*.

One may conduct this remembrance in thought or word and at any time. However, the Sufis have evolved certain congregational practices for this, which have come to mean the sitting in the circle of *dhikr*. It is perhaps this practice that has gained more attention than all other activities of the Sufis in various parts of the world.

The Prophet (s.a.w.s.) gave an account of what transpires in the congregation of *dhikr*.

The Holy Prophet (s.a.w.s.) has said that a group of angels is given a special duty by Allah to perform a patrol of the entire earth, looking for those who are engaged in remembrance of Allah the Almighty, chanting His name. When such assemblies are discovered, the angels are so amazed and pleased that they call more angels to join them and, placing their wings together in embrace, they make a column that reaches up into the Heavens.

When the assembly of *dhikr* has ended, these angels return to Heaven, and Allah asks them where they have been. (Even though He is already aware of what has transpired, He is pleased to hear of it.)

The angels tell Him that they are returning from an assembly of persons engaged in remembrance of Him and that they were glorifying and praising Him. Allah asks the angels, "Have they seen Me?" The angels reply, "No, Lord, they have not." Allah the Almighty then asks the angels, "What would those people think if they had seen Me?" The angels reply that in such a case, they would have been engaging themselves even more in His worship.

"What do they ask of Me?" Allah the Almighty then asks. "They long for Your Paradise," the angels respond. "Have they seen My Paradise?" Allah asks. "No, they have not seen it," the angels respond. "What would happen if they had seen it?" Allah inquires of the angels. "They would long for it all the more," is their reply.

Then Allah the Almighty asks the angels, "From what were the people seeking protection?" The angels inform Him that the people were seeking protection from the hell. "Have they seen My hell?" Allah inquires. "No, Lord, they have not," the angels reply. "What if they had seen My hell?" Allah the Almighty asks of the angels, who reply that the people would have even more sought refuge and protection from it.

Then Allah the Almighty commands each of the angels present that He has forgiven all of those who were engaged in remembrance of Him. One angel says to Allah, "But Lord, there was one among them who only accidentally sat down and did not belong there" (that is, he was insincere). Allah the Almighty replies, "Even that one have I forgiven, so exalted is the assembly that even one on the edge is not deprived of My reward."

The *dhikr* assembly takes many forms and is called *dhikr-ḥalqah, samā^{c}*, or simply *dhikr*. Each Sufi order may have its particular form and sequence of performing the *dhikr*, but these differences are so minor as to be inconsequential. The *dhikr* ceremony of the Chishti is composed of four parts, each lasting approximately one hour, although the shaykh present may extend the ceremony to five or more hours, depending upon the stations of those present. Pir Syed Daoud Iqbali, leader of the Naqshbandiyyah Sufis of Afghanistan, once remarked that any *dhikr* that lasts less than four or five hours is just "fooling around."

For anyone seriously interested in deriving the ultimate benefits of the Sufi *dhikr*, a true shaykh (or *murshid*) is an absolute necessity. As the one of the great Sufis commented: "He who has no shaykh and follows himself has taken satan as his guide."

Furthermore, Allah has warned us in the Qur'an that one who has no *murshid* becomes totally lost.

Generally, the *dhikr* ceremony is held on Thursday evening, which the Sufis consider the beginning of Friday, the day of community prayers in Islam. Usually the dervishes will arrive for dinner or shortly thereafter and pray the final night prayer (^{c}*ishā*) together. Then they await the signal from the shaykh to begin.

The seated dervishes form a circle, and the shaykh begins by reciting praises upon the Prophet Muhammad (s.a.w.s.) and various other supplications. Then the sacred formula of *La ilāha illā Llāhū* is intoned. This recitation follows the lead proposed by the shaykh. It may be swift or slow, loud or soft. In any event, the real object of the *dhikr*—intense as it may be—is not to get "high" or to become disoriented; rather, it is to ascend the ladder of stations of the soul, so that one may arrive at the Threshold and attain a glimpse of the Divine. When this happens (which is by no means uniformly achieved), the person may fall into a state of *wajd* (ecstasy). As a mark of respect, all present rise until this condition departs the dervish.

The shaykh signals the end of one phase of the *dhikr* and the beginning of the next. In the Chishtiyyah, the initial phase of the *dhikr* consists of recitation of *Lā ilāha illā Llāhū*, with a breath break at a particular place. The second, third, and fourth parts of the *dhikr* are composed of segments of the sacred formula (*illā Llāhū*, nothing except Allah; *Allāh*, God; and *Hū*, the One). Amendments to the *dhikr* may be made at the discretion of the shaykh, by adding various of the divine attributes (*ṣifāt*) at various places in the *dhikr*.

After the term of the *dhikr*, long or short, the shaykh or other dervish recites from the Holy Qur'an. There then follows extended supplications for the Prophet Muhammad (s.a.w.s.), his family and followers (may Allah have mercy on them all), the other prophets (a.s.), the pious ancestors in the order, and others.

The posture and motions of the head are done in a specific manner by the Sufi orders and constitutes the main differences among them.

In the Chishtiyyah Order, the *dhikr* is ordinarily accomplished in the following manner:

Lā ilāha illā Llāhū: First one must have ablution. Begin in a sitting posture as in prayer, the legs folded under the body. If the legs are crossed tailor-style, the vein in the juncture of the left leg behind the knee must be grasped with the big toe. This posture dispels evil insinuations and also dissolves fat around the area of the heart, which is the abode of the "sneaking whisperer" (*al-khannās*), one of the forms of the Devil.

While reciting, the head is moved in the motion of an arc, starting with the left cheek resting upon the left shoulder. The head is then swung downward across the chest, and a pause is made with the face looking upward. This is done as *Lā ilāha* is uttered. Then, as the syllable *ill* is voiced, the head is thrown rather forcefully downward in the direction of the heart. The recitation concludes by raising the head again, looking upward as "*Allāhū*" is said. These motions are summarized in the accompanying illustrations.

There is no harm if one takes up this practice in moderation—a few dozen times—alone. However, the Sufis have organized their students into the *tariqats*, so that close supervision can be maintained over those performing the various practices. Whenever making recitation of formulas to treat disease, it is important that the number of recitations end in zero (e.g., 30, 60, 100, 300). This is so because the desire is for the result to end with nothing.

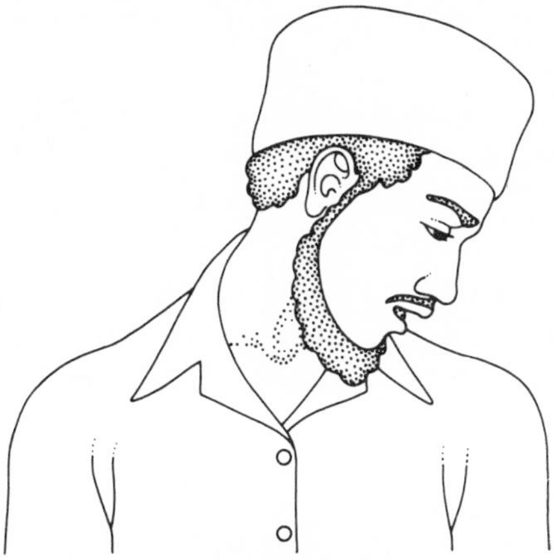

Initial head position,
Lā

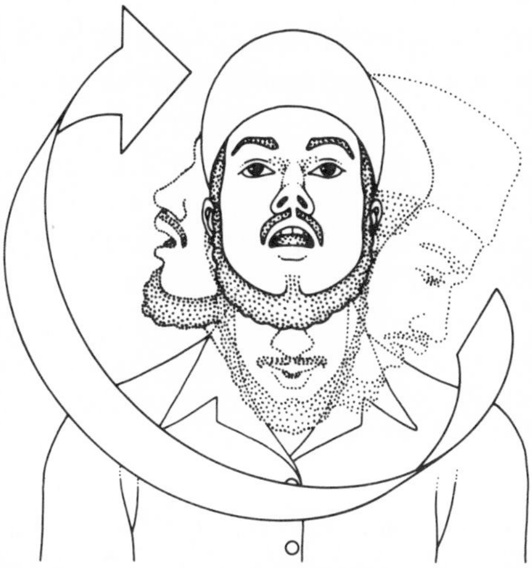

Second position,
ilāha

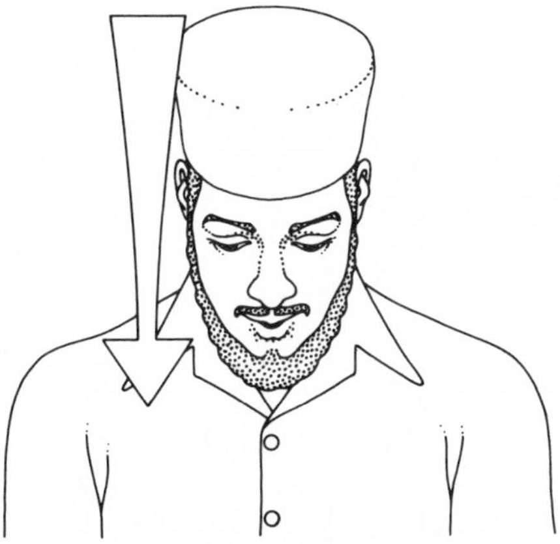

Third position,
ill

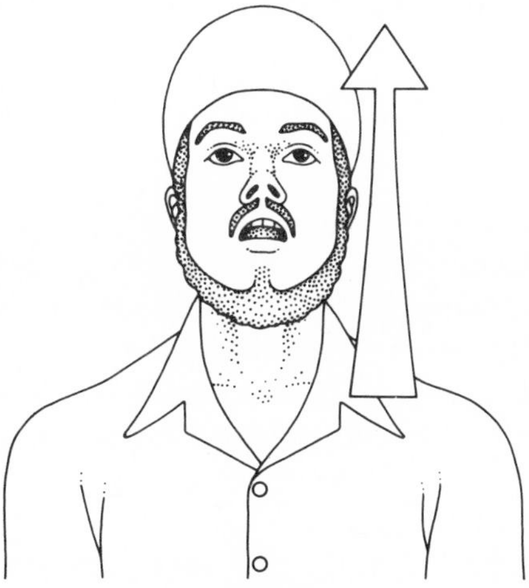

Fourth position,
Allāhū

As blithe as people may wish to be about taking up practices on their own, at the least severe mental confusions can result, and at the worst deaths have occurred.

The reason the *dhikr* is so effective is that the long vowel sounds of the words *Lā ilāha illā Llāhū* are primarily resonating in the heart, causing a tremendous dissemination of divine attributes in a very short time. Moreover, the breath is compressed and condensed in a manner that generates a high degree of heat, which itself burns out many physical impurities in the body. It is common to see dervishes drenched in sweat at the conclusion of the ceremony.

It is sometimes permitted to conduct short *dhikr* ceremonies without having a shaykh present. However, true dervishes always prefer to have one or more shaykhs present, owing to the channeling of *barakah*, or divine blessing, which only the shaykhs can accomplish.

I once attended a *dhikr* in the northern part of Afghanistan. About forty men were present. This particular Sufi order had conducted *dhikr* ceremonies every Thursday evening for almost 1,200 years without one interruption. *Mā shā' Allāh.*

As we were seated and beginning the initial recitations, the shaykh paused for a few seconds, and a loud grinding and whooshing sound roared through the adobe room. As I looked up, I perceived that a cleft had appeared in the far wall of the room, which sealed up in an instant. Later, at the end of the *dhikr*, the shaykh spent almost an hour reciting *salāms* of greeting to all of the pious souls who had slipped in through that cleft. *Yā Allāh!*

The shaykhs also advise and conduct another form of remembrance, which utilizes one or more of the ninety-nine divine attributes. These ninety-nine attributes are reproduced in Appendix III.

Not all of these attributes are used at all times. In the Chishtiyyah Order, five of these attributes have special significance and power. The specific attributes and the manner of utilizing them cannot be stated here. But to recite them in a particular manner, so many times, will convey the following effects: (1) prevent any enemy from doing any harm to one; (2) bring any sum of money desired; (3) compel everyone to treat one with kindness and to do any helpful thing; (4) remove all anxiety from the heart; and (5) end any disagreement or quarrel between two people. Such powers clearly must be guarded and preserved from falling into the hands of people of bad intentions.

I have seen many serious diseases driven out from those who sat among the circle of *dhikr*—and these people attempted no other treatment. The nature of Allah is not one of limitation or sickness, and one who fills the mind and heart with thought and consciousness of Allah will find that all things other than Allah are vanquished.

The *dhikr* accomplishes the following: drives away evil forces and defeats them; pleases Allah the Almighty; attracts livelihood; makes the personality impressive and prestigious; gives access to Allah the Almighty; revives and resuscitates the heart; banishes flaws and faults; saves the speech from gossip and backbiting; remedies all ailments of the heart; removes all fear and fright from the heart; prohibits hypocrisy.

Moreover, there exists one corner of the heart (and therefore certain divine potentialities within) that is not opened except by *dhikr*.

Dhikr of Allah the Almighty is the touchstone of all mystical practices of all Sufi orders. When one arrives at the state of performance of *dhikr*, with sincerity, one is at that famous stage when knowledge gleaned from books is of no further use. Allowed to flourish and unfold, the *dhikr* leads one, as He may decide, to the highest stages of human evolution, and one gains access to the origin of miracles.

ALLĀHŪ! ALLĀHŪ! ALLĀHŪ!

14

The Origin of Miracles

But His command,
when He intendeth a thing,
is only that He saith unto it:
Be! and it is.

Qur'an 36:82

A miracle is an event that happens outside of natural laws and beyond the ability of the human mind and reason to explain it. There are two words that mean "miracle" in Sufi healing, and the distinction between them is very important to understand. The first word is *mu^{c}jizah*, which refers to an intervention directly by God Himself in human and natural laws. The second word is *karāmah*, which means the use of a human as agency for a divine intervention. The distinction may seem subtle. The *mu^{c}jizah* may be any action that no human has requested or has any hand in its doing. For example, the virgin conception by Mary, mother of Jesus (a.s.), was a *mu^{c}jizah* of Allah, exalted is He. An example of a *karāmah* would be the raising of the dead body by Hazrat Jesus on his own command. However, in *both* cases, it is actually the power of Allah that causes these things to occur.

Abdullah Yusuf Ali (may Allah be pleased with him), writing in his commentary on the Holy Qur'an, said: "It is the privilege of the men of Allah to see the sublimest mysteries of the spiritual world and instruct men in righteousness; they warn and shield men against evil. But nothing can lessen each soul's responsibility for its own deeds. Each one carries his fate around his neck. Allah's gifts are for all, but not all receive the same gifts, nor are all gifts of equal dignity or excellence."

The Holy Prophet (s.a.w.s.), speaking of the type of person whom Allah favors with these mysteries, said: "Verily, Allah Most High hath a wine that He prepared for His friends [*awliyā'*]; when they drink it they are purified, and when they are purified they become nimble, and when they become nimble they soar, and when they soar they reach, and when they reach they unite, and when they unite they separate, and when they separate they pass away, and when they pass away they abide, and when they abide they become kings; then they are in the Assembly of Truth in the presence of a Sovereign Omnipotent."

The venerable shaykh al-Ḥabīb (r.a.) says of man, "If he but knew the secret of his mystery, he would shed a tear with every breath he breathed. . . ."

Accounts of the lives of Sufis are full of descriptions of what we would call miraculous experiences—travel into space, raising of the dead, healing the sick and other phenomena. Of course, the most impressive account is the ascension into heaven by the Prophet Muhammad (s.a.w.s.). During that visit, he learned many divine mysteries and met with the souls of many prophets and holy people, and he received instructions from Allah the Almighty Himself.

Hazrat Ibn ᶜArabī (r.a.), the great Sufi theologian of some eight centuries ago, reported visiting the moon and wrote out extensive accounts of characteristics of the environment to be found there—all of which was only recently confirmed by U.S. space explorers.

When he was but a child of six years old, Hazrat Mawlānā Rūmī (r.a.) terrified his playmates by leaping up into the sky and disappearing for an afternoon, while he was taken on a tour of the zodiacal constellations.

Such accounts may seem phenomenal, but they have occurred with such frequency and with so many eyewitnesses that they cannot be discounted simply because science at present may lack understanding of them.

Consider the existence of radio waves. For many thousands of years such waves have existed, but only in this century has man been able to identify, measure, and use them. The divine realities extend far beyond the capacity of the mind to view them, and humans can only glimpse these things when Allah allows it.

To the average person, miracles seem incomprehensible. However, ineffable as miracles are, they are real. One may legitimately wonder how miracles occur.

The *muᶜjizah*s, or direct miracles of Allah, are not so difficult to understand. When we realize that God created the entire universe and a great deal more, we should not falter in allowing any action to be within His capacity. However, when we hear of humans effecting such things, we are skeptical, Sufi or no! An analogy from our present society may cast some light on this complex and unfathomable subject.

We all use the telephone to reach across vast distances. By means of this rather simple device, we can dial a number of seven digits and reach another person in any part of our city. By adding just three more digits, we can reach anyone in the country. And just a few more numbers expands our reach to the world. People do this all the time. By using the telephone with a computer, the possibilities are greatly enlarged, and one can set in motion vastly complicated procedures. For example, if one had the knowledge of the correct numerical sequence, one could transfer millions of dollars from one bank account to another, even accounts thousands of miles away. Yet, if you presented the same fifteen-digit number to a person who did not possess the correct access code, nothing would happen. In a sense, what the Sufi does to instigate miracles, is analogous to the computer's work.

Allah the Almighty has said that the Qur'an is the Book of Guidance; moreover, He has said that there nothing is left out of the Qur'an. This claim may seem overdrawn to some, but it is true, on the authority of the Lord of the Worlds.

The shaykhs have recounted that each verse, or *ayat*, of the Qur'an has at least 18,000 meanings. Obviously, the human mind cannot affix 18,000 meanings to each verse. What this means is that there are in each *ayat* a vast number of meanings, which are perceived on unseen and unknown levels—the cellular, atomic, and subatomic levels—in ways that present technology and insight cannot witness or measure.

We have reviewed some of the considerations of vowel sounds and vibratory effects in reciting the Holy Qur'an. But each letter of the Arabic alphabet is assigned a relationship between the divine realm and the human world. The following list reveals the correspondence between each letter of the Arabic alphabet and the regions of the hierarchy of the universe.

alif (a) = **1** = ***al-Bāri'***: the Creator

bā (*b*) = **2** = ***al-ᶜaql***: Intellect

jīm (*j*) = **3** = ***an-nafs***: Soul

dāl (*d*) = **4** = ***aṭ-ṭabī'ah***: Nature

hā (*h*) = **5** = ***al-Bāri' bil-iḍāfah***: Creator in relation to what is below Him

waw (*w*) = **6** = ***al-ᶜAql bil-iḍāfah***: Intellect in relation to what is below it

zā' (*z*) = **7** = ***an-nafs bil-iḍāfah***: Soul in relation to what is below it

ḥā (*ḥ*) = **8** = ***aṭ-ṭabī'ah bil-idafah***: Nature in relation to what is below it

ṭā (*ṭ*) = **9** = ***al-hayūlā***: Material world, having no relation to anything below it

yā' (*y*) = **10** = ***al-ibdā'***: Plan of the Creator

kāf (*k*) = **20** = ***at-takwīn***: Structure transmitted to the created realm

lām (*l*) = **30** = ***al-amr***: The Divine Commandment (*kun fa-yakūn*)

mīm (*m*) = **40** = ***al-khalq***: The created universe

nūn (*n*) = **50** = ***al-wujūd***: The twofold aspect of being

sīn (*s*) = **60** = The doubled relation between *khalq* and *takwīn*

ᶜayn (ᶜ) = **70** = ***al-tarṭīb***: The chain of commands being impressed upon the universe

ṣād (ṣ) = **90** = The tripled relation between *amr, khalq,* and *takwīn*

qāf (*q*) = **100** = ***ijtimāl al-jumlah fil-ibdā'***: The assembly of all things in the plan of the Creator

rā (*r*) = **200** = ***at-tawhid***: Unity, the return of all things to the One, which is their principle and reason for existence

By assigning these cosmic values to each letter of the word *Allāh,* it can now be stated that certain events are being activated in the unseen realms, as follows:

ALLĀH

A = The Creator (the absolute Owner of all existence)
L = The divine commandment
H = Creator in relation to what is below Him (the divine essence [*dhāt*] in relation to His manifestations['*asmā'*])

To say the word *Qur'an* similarly invokes overtones in the divine realms:

AL-QŪR'AN

A = The Creator (the absolute Owner of all existence)
L = The divine commandment
Q = The assembly of all things in the plan of the Creator (the final code covering and ordering all of existence)
R = The return of all things to the One (the divine purpose in creation)
A = Creator, Who by ordering sets in motion the foregoing Intention
N = The twofold aspect of being (the separation from the Creator: man and God)

Thus, for the Sufi, when the word *Allah* is spōken, a sequence of stirrings are ignited within the deepest recesses of his mind and soul, which remind (*dhikr*) the rememberer of the One remembered.

The very essence of the human being, when saying the word *Allāh,* is impressed in this manner: the Creator, the Absolute Lord and Master of all existence, in sending a soul into human life, imbues the soul with an inherent knowledge of and obedience to the divine commandments. These exist and are interwoven in an inexpressibly refined manner within the body/mind/soul of the human being. Then the Creator issues the order to the soul to inhabit a particular drop of sensitized blood (ovum), and life begins. From that moment, human life is nothing except a reflection of the Creator.

A similar soliloquy is suggested with the word *Qur'an*: The Book, *al-Kitab.*

The Qur'an is the collection of the information of "all things in the plan of the Creator." Allah has said that nothing has been left out of the Qur'an, and that if all the trees were pens and all the oceans ink, and all of this doubled, we could not write down the knowledge contained in the Qur'an.

With the utterance of the first letter of the Qur'an, we are stirring within the deepest parts of our mental and psychological world. As we continue the word, making the sound of the letter *rā*, our souls are beckoned to the return of all things to the One." As the first three letters ignite the unimaginably immense totality of the Plan of the Creator and our purpose in human life, the fourth letter, *alif*, stirs again remembrance of the Creator, declaring the reality of our present situation of duality, of separation and absence of union with our Lord. Indeed this is the eternal condition of life. This is not an idea.

The science of Sufism is conducted within a closed society, an esoteric, private group. The knowledge possessed by the Sufis is derived from the deep immersions in the nature of existence referred to above. Allah has provided the"access codes" to utilize these knowledges to effect miracles on the human plane.

Examples have been given of reciting a particular divine attribute a particular number of times, to prevent harm from one's enemy. Other codes exist to utilize a great many *ayats* of the Qur'an. (The word *ayat*, incidentally, means both "verse" and "miracle.") One Sufi practice creates an effect upon the soul equal to performance of *salat* for seven hundred years. The practice itself requires only about five seconds of recitation. Now, not everyone could endure such a practice. For some, it would be like giving a full syringe of penicillin to a fly suffering from a cold!

By adding practices together, the effects are extended to a point that they cannot be expressed even using mathematical abstract concepts. Some Sufis have accomplished recitations of these formulas running into the tens of millions of times.

One of the problems of expressing concepts of Sufi healing is that one who may witness a healing, even a miraculous one, can perceive very little going on. Someone appears before the shaykh, the shaykh seems to mumble something and blows a breath toward the patient, and the patient is healed of a crippling disease. Yet one cannot witness the decades of preparation required for the shaykh to perform that act. It may have been that the shaykh sat in seclusion for thirty years, reciting a formula fifty million times, to be able to heal that one person. And that healing may have been the shaykh's main purpose in life.

Some people would like the Sufis to provide a list of diseases and the specific formulas that would miraculously cure them. However, it is not the formula per se but the utilization of the formula by means of the agency of the purified breath and soul of the shaykh that causes the effects. The formulas by themselves would be rather useless to the lay person.

The human mind and body become clouded and covered over with impurities, making the exercise of true reason difficult. In addition to these impurities, the influence of various societal and familial indoctrinations ultimately succeed in making a human being a mere shadow of the exalted and majestic being that the God the Most High granted as each person's birthright.

It requires a vast and difficult blend of medications to cleanse the conditions of those in states of imbalance. No two illnesses are exactly the same, so the remedies must be formulated individually for each person, with attention to harmonizing the treatments for body, mind, and soul. The objective of the Sufi shaykh, as physician, is not merely to relieve a person of some physical pain or inconvenience, but to see a total reformation of each person's life in accord with the Divine Blessings and plan of the Creator, exalted is He.

Sufi Barkat Ali (may Allah grant him the choicest blessings, as many of such things as there are) once remarked: "Only hearts can impart knowledge about hearts. And this knowledge is bestowed, not acquired."

Initially these assertions may have to be taken on faith. But anyone who cares to put them to the test will find that faith transformed into belief, *in shā' Allāh*.

The final chapters of this book present several practices that are highly charged with divine grace and blessings. One of these practices has, as only one of its effects, the protection against any disease for the day one performs it. The second practice is known to cure any disease.

Yā Hayyu! Yā Qayyūm!

15

The Keys of the Treasures of the Heavens and the Earth

If ye count the favors of Allah,
Never will ye be able to number them.

Qur'an 14:33

Some of the concepts and ideals expressed in the preceding pages may be difficult for the novice to apply. However, the practice I shall present now can be done easily by anyone and encompasses all of the material that has been presented thus far. As far as I am aware, this is the first presentation of this practice of the Sufis to a general audience in the West.

A prerequisite for any Sufi healing formula to work is a particular recitation. Therefore, the following profession is provided, which will open the gates of the oceans of Mercy of Allah the Almighty, *insha Allah*. The formula is:

Lā ilāha illā Llāh; Muḥammadun Rasūlu Llāh.

This profession should be recited once before attempting any Sufi practice, lest malevolent forces be brought into play. It is also wise to utter the verse that seals off any satanic participation, as follows:

A^{c}ūdhu bi-Llāhi min ash-shayṭān ir-rajīm.

If you are unacquainted with the Arabic language, read the transliterations carefully and try and say the words as best as you can—and hope that you have said it correctly.

Although there are thousands of prayers, supplications, and practices used by the Sufis, several are considered to be superior. Such is the one here presented, called Maqalad as-Samawati wal Ard, the Keys of the Treasures of the Heavens and the Earth. Although it is specific to healing—conveying protection against any illness for the day it is recited—the benefits attached to its recitation are not limited to physical health, as one can glean for the following account from the Hadith:

It is reported that ^{c}Uthmān ibn ^{c}Affān, may Allah be pleased with him, requested further information about Allah's injunction of the Keys of the Treasures of the Heavens and the Earth (mentioned several times in the Qur'an). The Prophet (s.a.w.s.) said to him: "You have inquired of me something which nobody has ever asked me before. The Keys of the Treasures of the Heavens and the Earth are as follows":

لَآ إِلٰهَ إِلَّا اللّٰهُ وَاللّٰهُ أَكْبَرُ
وَسُبْحَانَ اللّٰهِ وَالْحَمْدُ لِلّٰهِ وَ
أَسْتَغْفِرُ اللّٰهَ الَّذِي لَآ إِلٰهَ إِلَّا
هُوَ الْأَوَّلُ وَالْآخِرُ وَالظَّاهِرُ
وَالْبَاطِنُ يُحْيِي وَيُمِيتُ وَهُوَ
حَيٌّ لَا يَمُوتُ بِيَدِهِ الْخَيْرُ
وَهُوَ عَلٰى كُلِّ شَيْءٍ قَدِيرٌ ۝

Lā ilāha illā Llāhu wa-Llāhu akbar.
Wa subḥān Allāhi wal-ḥamdu li-Llāhi
wastaghfiru Llāh alladhī lā ilāha illā Hū
wal-Awwalu wal-Ākhiru waẓ-Ẓāhiru wal-Bāṭinu
yuḥyi wa yumītu wa huwa Ḥayyan lā yamūtu.
Bi-yadihil-khayr wa huwa ^{c}alā kulli shay'in Qadīr.

There is none worthy of worship except Allah.
Allah the Almighty is the greatest.
Allah is the glorious and praiseworthy
and I ask Allah for forgiveness.
There is no power to do good
and no strength to be saved from evil
except with the grace of Allah.
He is the First and the Last.
He is the Apparent and the Hidden.
He is the Ever-Living Who never dies.
He imparts and takes away life.
There is blessing with Allah the Almighty.
He is the Ruler over everything.

The Prophet (s.a.w.s.) continued: "O ᶜUthmān! Whoever recites it one hundred times every day will be rewarded by ten graces. First, all his previous sins will be forgiven. Second, his suffering from hellfire will be written off. Third, two angels are appointed to guard him day and night from his sufferings and diseases. Fourth, he is granted a treasure of blessings. Fifth, he will reap as much blessing as someone who would have set free one hundred slaves from the offspring of the prophet Ishmael (a.s.). Sixth, he would be rewarded of blessings as if he had read the entire Qur'an, the Psalms, the Torah, and the Bible. Seventh, a house will be constructed for him in the Heaven. Eighth, he will be married to a pious Heavenly maiden. Ninth, he will be honored with a crown of honor. Tenth, his recommendation (for forgiveness) of seventy of his relatives will be accepted.

"O ᶜUthmān! If you were strong enough you would not miss this remembrance on any day. You will be one of the successful ones and you will surpass everybody before and after you."

One of the great contemporary Sufis, Hazrat Abu Anees Barkat Ali of Dar-ul-Ehsan, Pakistan, has achieved a unique position among the men of piety by reciting this sacred formula. He has erected a large signpost at the entranceway of his spiritual sanctuary, upon which the words of this invaluable formula are inscribed. His own life bears ample testament to the efficacy of these words, as he has personally adopted more than ten thousand Hindus of the lowest caste and provided them with a complete training and education in life. Moreover, he maintains a clinic that provides medical care and that has restored the sight of more than three thousand persons so far, without charge of any kind. He has written more than three hundred books on Islam and Sufism, all of which have been distributed free of charge (the jacket of one reads: "These books are written for ourselves and you to read, but not for sale. They have already been sold to Him for Whom they were meant"). A countless stream of devotees arrive at the well-known Dar-ul-Ehsan sanctuary and receive, by His grace, spiritual instructions from among the fourteen Sufi orders of which Barkat Ali is a teaching master, or shaykh. *Mā shā' Allāh!* The qualities and attributes of Sufi Barkat Ali could be enumerated further, but anyone who views his life with an open mind must conclude that he has exceeded the usual range of human accomplishments. He is now in his seventy-sixth year.

The formula for the Keys of the Treasures of the Heavens and the Earth may be recited twenty-one times after each daily prayer and requires not more than three or four minutes to do so.

As Allah says: "As for those who strive in Us, surely We guide them to Our paths" (Qur'an 29:69).

On the night of fifth Rajab, A.H. 633, the great saint Hazrat Khwāja Muᶜīnuddīn Chishtī (r.a.) as usual retired to his meditation cell after the night prayer (*ᶜishā*). He closed the door and commenced his practice, as he had done for the past thirty years, of constant and incessant recitation of the above verses. The Khwāja instructed his *murīd*s not to disturb him that night. They stayed away, but heard through the door a sound expressing unparalleled ecstasy throughout the night. In the early hours of the morning, this sound ceased. When the door of his cell did not open at the time of morning prayers (*fajr*), anxiety was felt by everyone. Ultimately, the door was forced open by his students, who, to their astonishment, found that the soul of the great saint had relinquished his mortal body. The following sentence was radiantly glittering upon his forehead, as light:

Hadhā habību Llāh
Māta fī hubbi Llāh

He is the beloved of Allah
And he died in Allah's Love.

16

The Infallible Remedy

Once I saw the Most High God
in a dream.
He asked me, "Bayazid, what do you
want?"
I replied, "I want what You want."
The Most High God was pleased
and said,
"I am yours and you are Mine."
Shaykh Bayazid Bistami (r.a.)

The Holy Prophet of Allah the Almighty (s.a.w.s.), whose virtues are the most excellent, was the most trustworthy person of all creation. Even prior to his mission as Prophet, he was called *Amīn*, the trustworthy, and was never known to have spoken anything except the truth.

The Prophet (s.a.w.s.) said: "In Sūrat al-Fātiḥah there is a balm for all ailments." He went on to provide the specific instructions for utilizing this most treasured remedy.

The Prophet (s.a.w.s.) also said: "I tell you of a *sūrah* that is the greatest, the most virtuous, in the Holy Qur'an. It is Sūrat al-Ḥamd [the opening sūrah, al-Fātiḥah], which has seven verses. These are the *sab^{c}ah mathānī* [the Oft-Repeated Seven] and represent the Grand Qur'an."

In another Hadith, the Prophet (s.a.w.s.) is reported to have said: "By Him Who is in possession of my life, a *sūrah* like this one has been revealed neither in the Torah nor in the Bible, nor even in the rest of the Qur'an."

The accumulated experience of the Sufis confirms that the reading and reciting of Sūrat al-Fātiḥah with true faith and sincere conviction, cures all maladies, whether spiritual or worldly, external or internal. The Sūrat al-Fātiḥah enters into the writing of almost all *ta^{c}widh*; it is also written in ink made of saffron and rose water, and consumed. All six books of authentic (*saḥīḥ*) Hadith report that the Companions (r.a.a.) used to read it for treatment of diseases, both physical and mental.

The satan lamented, wept, and tore his hair out on four occasions: when

المنزل ١

بِسْمِ اللَّهِ الرَّحْمَٰنِ الرَّحِيمِ ①

الْحَمْدُ لِلَّهِ رَبِّ الْعَالَمِينَ ②

الرَّحْمَٰنِ الرَّحِيمِ ③

مَالِكِ يَوْمِ الدِّينِ ④

إِيَّاكَ نَعْبُدُ وَإِيَّاكَ نَسْتَعِينُ ⑤

اهْدِنَا الصِّرَاطَ الْمُسْتَقِيمَ ⑥

صِرَاطَ الَّذِينَ أَنْعَمْتَ عَلَيْهِمْ غَيْرِ الْمَغْضُوبِ

ع عَلَيْهِمْ وَلَا الضَّالِّينَ ⑦

Bismi Llāh ir-Raḥmān ir-Raḥīm
Il-ḥamdu li-Llāhi rabb il-^{c}ālāmin
Ar-raḥmān ir-Raḥīm
Māliki yawm id-dīn.
Iyyāka na^{c}budu wa iyyāka nasta^{c}īn.
Ihdinaṣ-ṣirāṭ al-mustaqīm
Ṣirāṭ alladhīna an^{c}amta ^{c}alayhim
Ghayril-maghḍūbi ^{c}alayhim wa lāḍ-ḍālīn.

1. In the Name of Allah, the Beneficent, the Merciful.
2. Praise be to Allah, Lord of the Worlds;
3. The Beneficent, the Merciful;
4. Master of the Day of Judgment!
5. Thee only do we worship;
Thee alone we ask for help.
6. Guide us on the straight path;
7. The path of those whom You love;
Not the path of those who earn Thine anger,
nor of those who go astray.

he was cursed, when he was thrown out of Heaven, when Muhammad (s.a.w.s.) was given Prophethood, and when Sūrat al-Fātiḥah was revealed.

Hazrat Khwāja Mu^{c}īnuddīn Chishtī (r.a.) has said, "The incessant recitation of Sūrat al-Fātiḥah is the infallible remedy for one's needs."

The recitation of Sūrat al-Fātiḥah is among the most frequent of the practices of the shaykhs of the path. The Prophet Muhammad (s.a.w.s.) suggested the following mode of recitation and said that this practice will succeed in curing any disease.

Read Sūrat al-Fātiḥah forty-one times for forty consecutive days, during the interval between the *sunnah* (optional) and *fard* (obligatory) *ra^{c}kat*s of the *fajr* (early-morning) prayer. In this recitation, it is necessary to *omit* the breath pause usually taken between the first two verses. In other words, the *mim* of *ir-Raḥīm* is joined with the *lam* of *al-ḥamdu li-Llāhi,* which then becomes *mil-ḥamdu li-Llāhi*. The rest of the *sūrah* may be done following the usual breath pauses.

If the person is possessed of madness, or for other reasons cannot perform the recitation, the words should be recited and blown on water, and given to the patient to drink.

We reproduce again Sūrat al-Fātiḥah on the facing page, for anyone who may wish to make use of its miraculous healing effects.

For some, even this recitation may prove to be difficult, or impossible for some reason or another. The mercy of Allah is infinite! If, after trying with absolute sincerity to learn and apply anything in this book, one fails to do so, the following will cure any disease. Simply recite eleven times: *Bismi Llāh ir-Raḥmān, ir-Raḥīm*. This verse is the Greatest Attribute of Allah the Almighty, and whatever endeavors to intrude upon the absolute sanctity of His grace is burnt to ashes.

Once Hazrat Abū Bakr (r.a.) was ill. The people came to visit him and seeing his obvious distress, asked him, "Why don't you call the doctor?" Abū Bakr answered, "I already called the doctor." His friend asked, "What did the doctor say?" Abū Bakr replied, "He said, 'I am Mighty in what I intend.'"

There is nothing that can defeat the love of Allah the Almighty for His beloved friends.

And after this, there remains nothing further that can, or should, be said.

Allāhu a^{c}lam!
As-salāmu ^{c}alaykum wa raḥmatu Llāhi wa barakatuhu!

Rabbi qad ātaytani min al-mulki
wa ^{c}allamtani min ta'wil il-ahādith
Fāṭir as-samāwāti wal-arḍ!
Anta walīyī fid-dunyā wal-ākhirah.
Tawaffanī musliman wa alhiqnī biṣ-ṣālihin.
Ashhadu an lā ilāha illā Llāh;
Wa ashhadu anna Muḥammadan ^{c}abduhu wa rasūluh. Āmīn!

O my Lord!
Thou hast given me something of sovereignty
and hast taught me something
of the interpretation of events—
Creator of the Heavens and the Earth!
Thou art my protecting Friend
in this world and the Hereafter.
Make me to die submissive unto Thee
and join me to the righteous.
I bear witness
that there is no deity except Allah
and I bear witness
That Muhammad is His servant and Messenger. Be it so!

As-salāmu ᶜalaykum wa raḥmatu Llāhi wa barakatuhu!

May the peace and blessings of God be upon you.

APPENDIXES

I
The Islamic Calendar

The Muslim year is based upon a lunar cycle of 354 days, consisting of 12 months of 29 or 30 days. This calendar commenced in the year 622 of the common era (C.E.), when the Prophet Muhammad (s.a.w.s.) migrated from Mecca to Medina. The 12 Islamic months are as follows.

Muḥarram: The 10th of this month is called ᶜAshurah, commemorating the martyrdom of Husayn ibn ᶜAlī, who died at Karbalah on the 10th Muḥarram 680 C.E.

Ṣafar

Rabīᶜ al-Awwal: The 12th of this month is the birthday of the Prophet Muhammad (s.a.w.s.).

Rabīᶜ ath-Thānī: The 11th of this month is the birthday of ᶜAbdul-Qādir Jīlānī (r.a.).

Jumādā al-Ūlā

Jumādā al-Ākhirah

Rajab: The 27th of this month is the anniversary of the *miᶜrāj*, the ascension of the Prophet (s.a.w.s.) to Heaven. The 6th of this month celebrates the death anniversary of Hazrat Khwāja Muᶜīnuddīn Chishtī (r.a.).

Shaᶜbān: The 14th–15th of this month is Shab al-Barā'at, when the destinies for the coming year are assigned.

Ramaḍān: The Sacred Month of Fasting. On either the 23rd, 25th, or 27th night, the Laylat al-Qadr (Night of Power) occurs. During this month, the Qur'an, as well as all other revealed books, first descended from Allah the Most High.

Shawwal: The first day is ᶜĪd al-Fiṭr, the feast celebrating the breaking of the fast.

Dhūl Qaᶜdah

Dhul-Hijjah: The pilgrimage to Mecca (*hajj*) is completed during this month. From the 10th to the 12th, the sacrifice of ᶜĪd al-Aḍḥā is celebrated.

As the dates are based upon lunar cycles and the sightings of the new moon, each year the calendar backs up by approximately eleven days.

II
Some Useful Short Sūrahs of the Holy Qur'an

112: Sūrat al-Ikhlāṣ (The Unity)

بِسْمِ اللَّهِ الرَّحْمَٰنِ الرَّحِيمِ ○

قُلْ هُوَ اللَّهُ أَحَدٌ ①

اللَّهُ الصَّمَدُ ②

لَمْ يَلِدْ وَلَمْ يُولَدْ ③

وَلَمْ يَكُن لَّهُ كُفُوًا أَحَدٌ ④ ٣٧

Bismi Llāh ir-Raḥmān ir-Raḥīm.

1. Qul Huwa Llāhu Aḥad;
2. Allāhuṣ-Ṣamad;
3. Lam yalid, wa lam yūlad;
4. Wa lam yakul lahū kufuwan aḥad.

In the name of Allah, the Beneficent, the Merciful.

1. Say: He is Allah, the One!
2. Allah the eternally besought of all!
3. He begetteth not nor was begotten
4. And there is none comparable to Him.

113: Sūrat al-Falaq (The Daybreak)

بِسْمِ اللَّهِ الرَّحْمَٰنِ الرَّحِيمِ

قُلْ أَعُوذُ بِرَبِّ الْفَلَقِ ﴿١﴾

مِن شَرِّ مَا خَلَقَ ﴿٢﴾

وَمِن شَرِّ غَاسِقٍ إِذَا وَقَبَ ﴿٣﴾

وَمِن شَرِّ النَّفَّاثَاتِ فِي الْعُقَدِ ﴿٤﴾

وَمِن شَرِّ حَاسِدٍ إِذَا حَسَدَ ﴿٥﴾

Bismi Llāh ir-Raḥmān ir-Raḥīm.

1. Qul a'ūdhu bi-rabb il-falaq.
2. Min sharri mā khalaq.
3. Wa min sharri ghāsiqin idhā waqab.
4. Wa min sharrin naffāthāti fīl-ᶜuqad,
5. Wa min sharri ḥāsidin idhā ḥasad.

In the name of Allah, the Beneficent, the Merciful.

1. Say: I seek refuge in the Lord of Daybreak
2. From the evil of that which He created.
3. From the evil of the darkness when it is intense,
4. And from the evil of malignant witchcraft,
5. And from the evil of the envier when he envieth.

114: Sūrat an-Nās (Mankind)

بِسْمِ اللّٰهِ الرَّحْمٰنِ الرَّحِيْمِ ○

قُلْ اَعُوْذُ بِرَبِّ النَّاسِ ﴿١﴾

مَلِكِ النَّاسِ ﴿٢﴾

اِلٰهِ النَّاسِ ﴿٣﴾

مِنْ شَرِّ الْوَسْوَاسِ الْخَنَّاسِ ﴿٤﴾

الَّذِيْ يُوَسْوِسُ فِيْ صُدُوْرِ النَّاسِ ﴿٥﴾

مِنَ الْجِنَّةِ وَالنَّاسِ ﴿٦﴾

Bismi Llāh ir-Raḥmān ir-Raḥīm.
1. Qul a'ūdhy bi-Rabbin-nās,
2. Mālikin-nās,
3. Ilāhin-nās
4. Min sharr il-waswās il-khannās,
5. Alladh-i yuwaswisu fi ṣudūrin-nāsi,
6. Min al-jinnati wan-nās.

In the name of Allah, the Beneficent, the Merciful.
1. Say: I seek refuge in the Lord of mankind,
2. The King of mankind,
3. The God of mankind.
4. From the evil of the Sneaking Whisperer,*
5. Who whispereth in the hearts of mankind,
6. Of the jinn and mankind.

*An epithet of Satan.

III
The Divine Attributes

Allah the Almighty is, in the end, unknowable. Regardless of how we may try, we are left with an incomplete and partial understanding of Him. *Allāhu akbar* is the frequent utterance of the Sufis. It means: "Allah is Greater than all that we ascribe to Him."

So that we may begin to have a mental concept of Him, Allah has set forth, in the Holy Qur'an, ninety-nine of His divine attributes. Considered together, they provide a concept of His all-encompassing, all-pervading, all-powerful nature. These attributes, called *al-asmā' al-ḥusnā* (The Beautiful Names), enter into Sufi practices called *waẓifah*s.

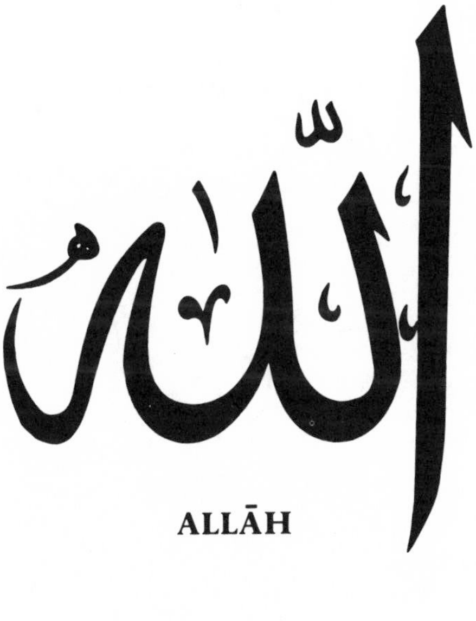

ALLĀH

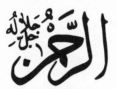

الرحمن جل جلاله

1. AR-RAḤMĀN
The Gracious;
The Beneficent;
The Compassionate

الرحيم جل جلاله

2. AR-RAḤĪM
The Merciful

الملك جل جلاله

3. AL-MALĪK
The King;
The Sovereign Lord

القدوس جل جلاله

4. AL-QUDDŪS
The Holy

السلام جل جلاله

5. AS-SALĀM
The Peace

المؤمن جل جلاله

6. AL-MU'MIN
The Keeper of Faith;
The Bestower of Security;
The Faithful

المهيمن جل جلاله

7. AL-MUHAYMIN
The Protector;
The Guardian

العزيز جل جلاله

8. AL-ᶜAZĪZ
The Mighty

الجبار جل جلاله

9. AL-JABBĀR
The Compeller

المتكبر جل جلاله

10. AL-MUTAKABBIR
The Majestic;
The Superb

الخالق جل جلاله

11. AL-KHĀLIQ
The Creator

البارئ جل جلاله

12. AL-BĀRI'
The Maker-out-of-Naught

المصور جل جلاله

13. AL-MUṢAWWIR
The Fashioner

الغفار جل جلاله

14. AL-GHAFFĀR
The Forgiver

القهار جل جلاله

15. AL-QAHHĀR
The Subduer;
The Almighty;
The Conquering

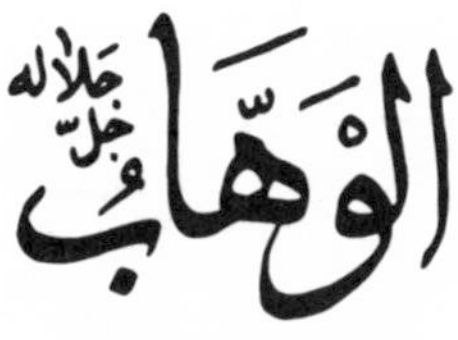

16. AL-WAHHĀB
The Bestower

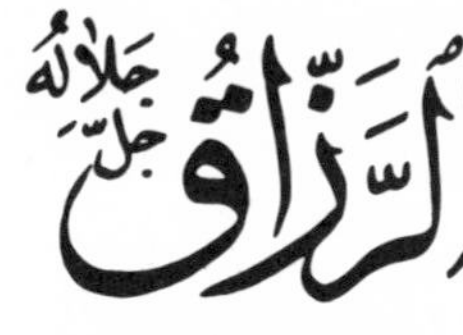

17. AR-RAZZĀQ
The Provider;
The Sustainer

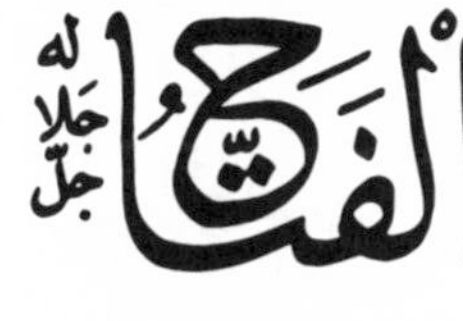

18. AL-FATTĀḤ
The Opener;
The Reliever;
The Judge

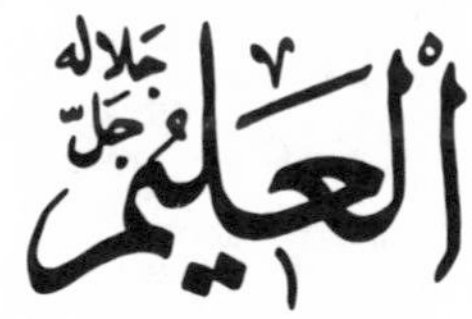

19. Al-ᶜALĪM
The All-Knowing;
The Knower

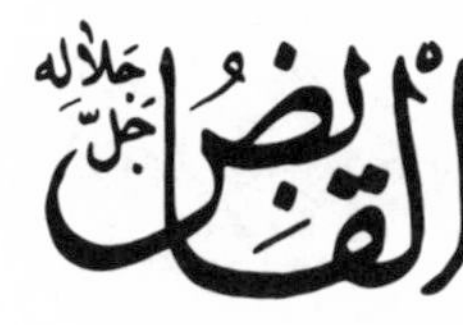

20. AL-QĀBIḌ
The Restrainer;
The Withholder

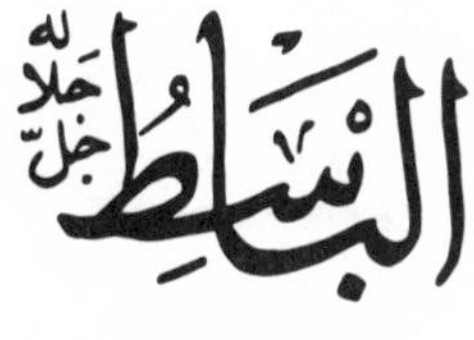

21. AL-BĀSIṬ
The Extender;
The Enlarger;
The Spreader

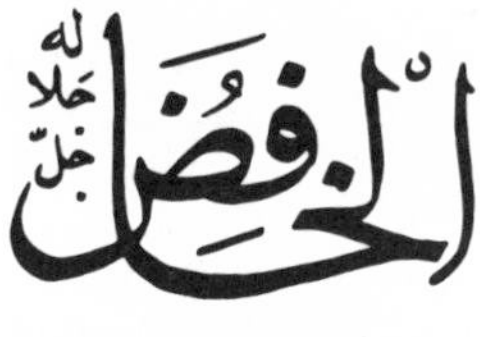

22. AL-KHĀFIḌ
The Abaser

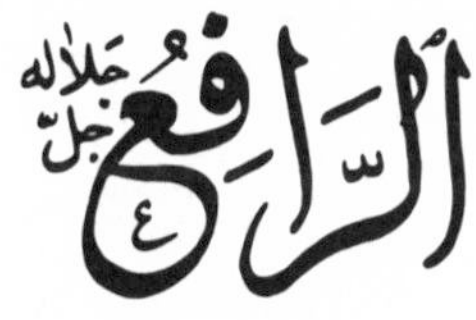

23. AR-RĀFIᶜ
The Exalter

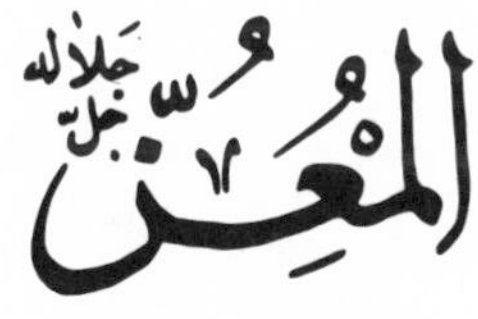

24. AL-MUᶜIZZ
The Honorer;
The Strengthener

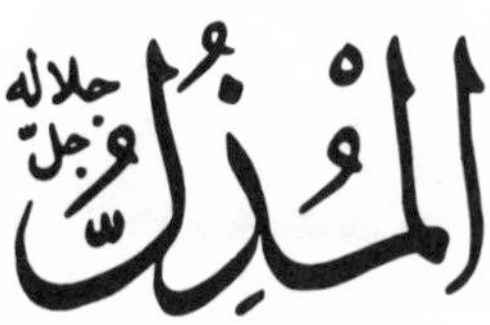

25. AL-MUDHILL
The Dishonerer;
The Humiliator

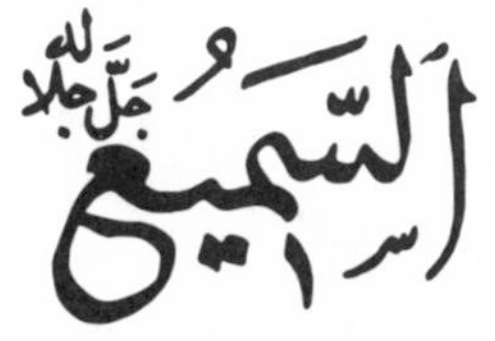

26. AS-SAMĪᶜ
The All-Hearing;
The Hearer

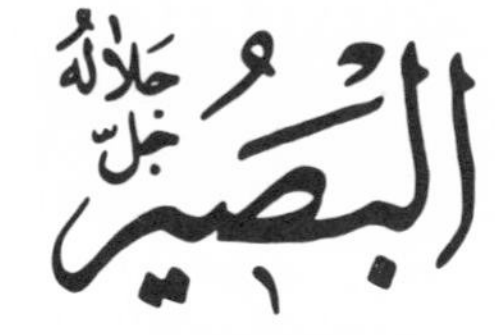

27. AL-BAṢĪR
The All-Seeing;
The Perceiver

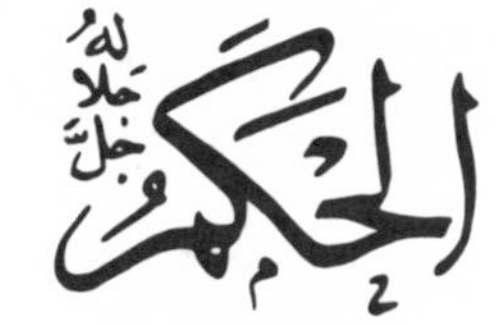

28. AL-ḤAKAM
The Judge

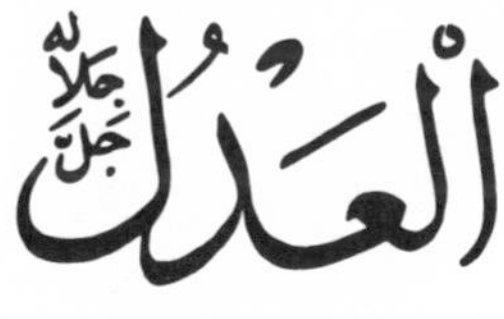

29. AL-ᶜADL
The Just;
The Equitable

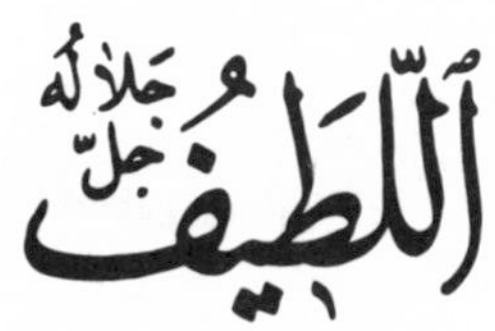

30. AL-LAṬĪF
The Subtle;
The Gracious

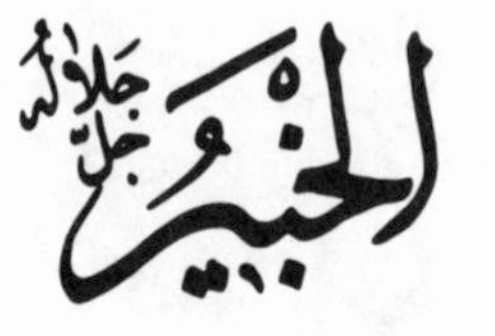

31. AL-KHABĪR
The Aware

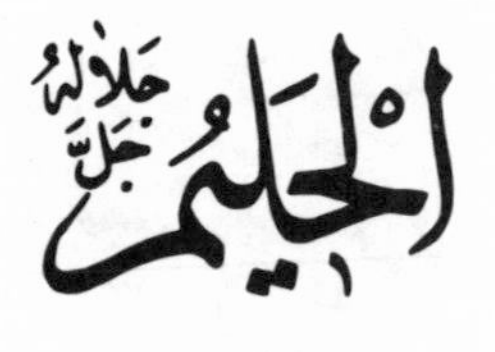

32. AL-ḤALĪM
The Forbearing;
The Clement

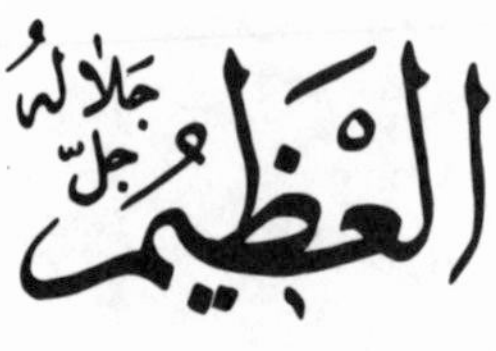

33. AL-^{C}AẒĪM
The Magnificent;
The Tremendous

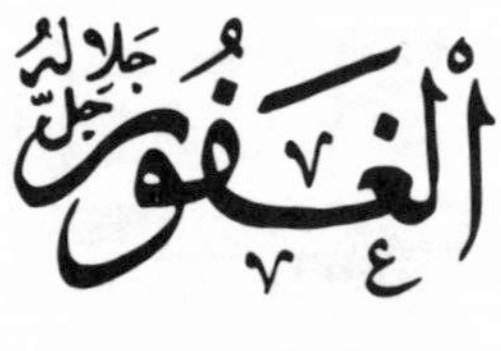

34. AL-GHAFŪR
The Forgiving

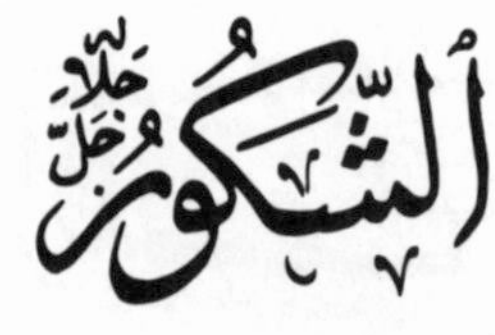

35. ASH-SHAKŪR
The Grateful;
The Repayer of Good

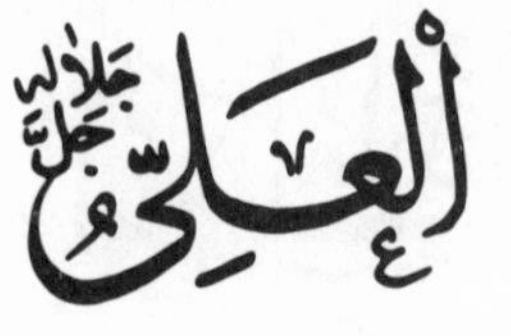

36. AL-^{C}ALĪ
The High;
The Sublime

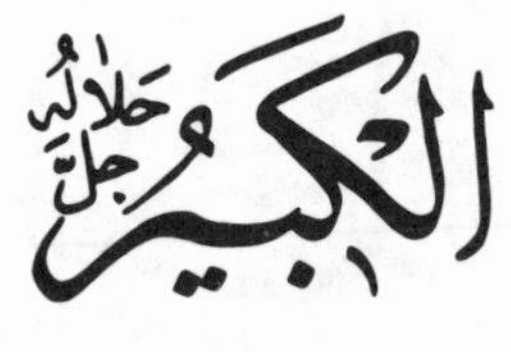

37. AL-KABĪR
The Great

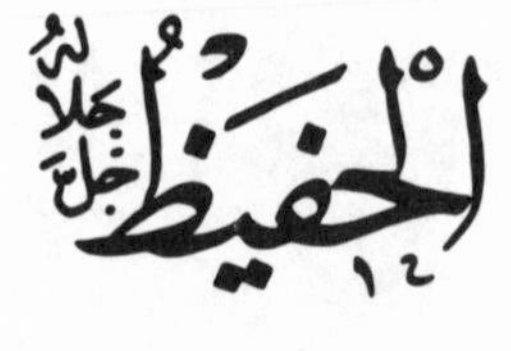

38. AL-ḤAFĪẒ
The Preserver;
The Protector;
The Guardian

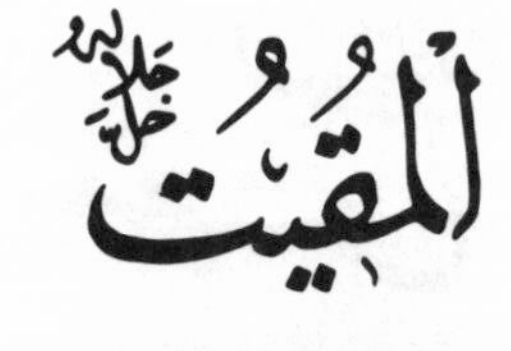

39. AL-MUQĪT
The Feeder;
The Sustainer;
The Strengthener

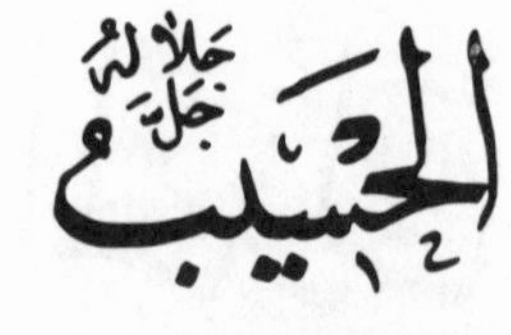

40. AL-ḤASĪB
The Reckoner

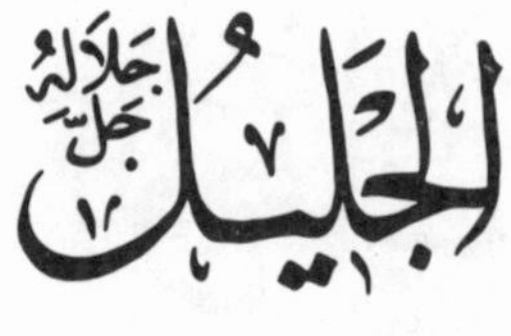

41. AL-JALĪL
The Majestic

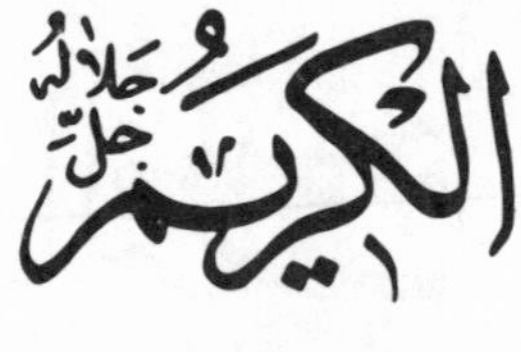

42. AL-KARĪM
The Bountiful;
The Generous

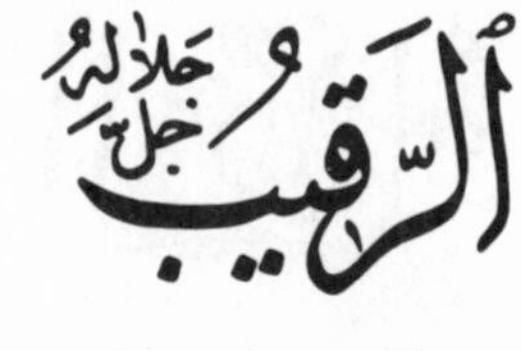

43. AR-RAQĪB
The Watcher;
The Watchful

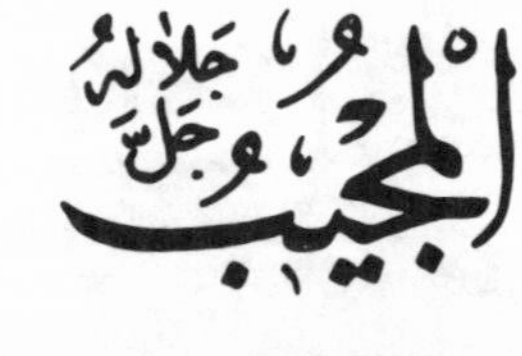

44. AL-MUJĪB
The Responsive;
The Hearkener
(to prayer)

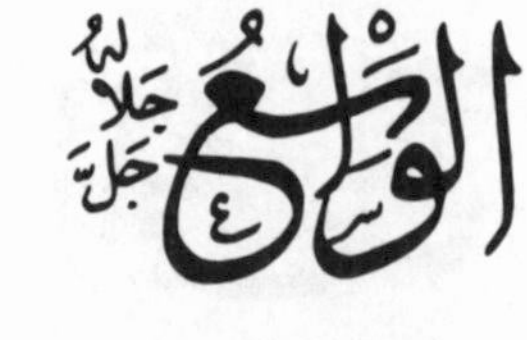

45. AL-WĀSI^{C}
The Vast;
The All-Embracing;
The Comprehensive

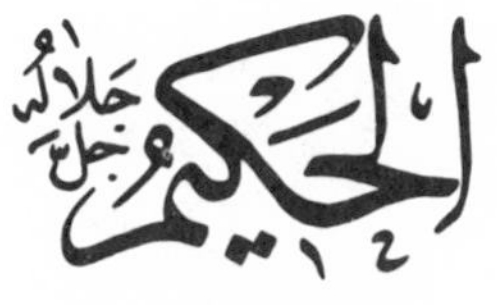

46. AL-ḤAKĪM
The Wise

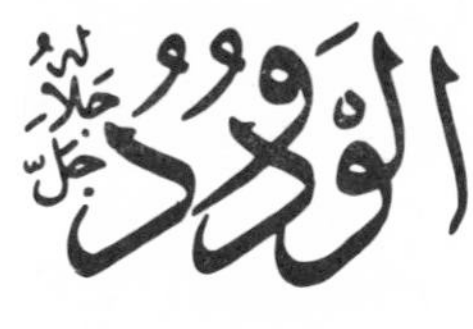

47. AL-WADŪD
The Loving

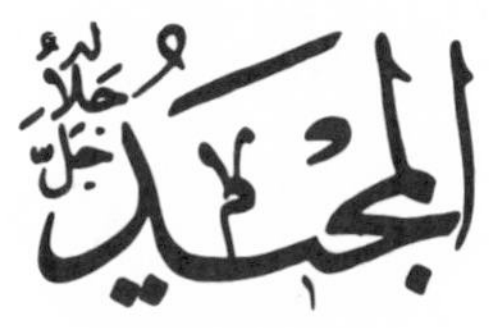

48. AL-MAJĪD
The Glorious

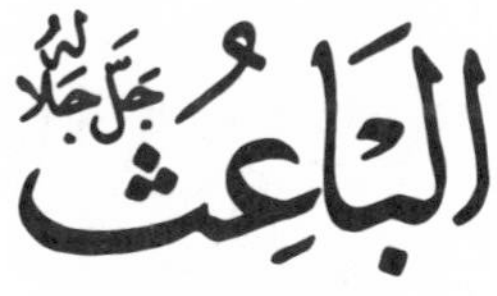

49. AL-BĀᶜITH
The Raiser (from death)

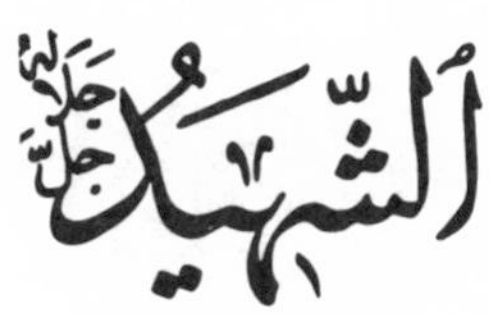

50. ASH-SHAHĪD
The Witness

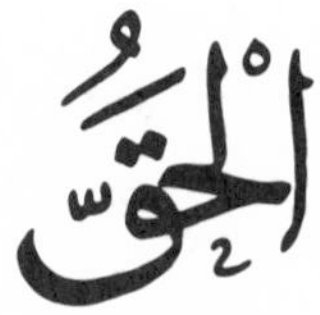

51. AL-ḤAQQ
The Truth

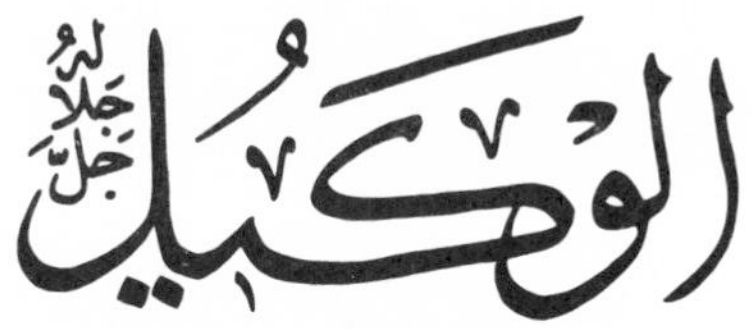

52. AL-WAKĪL
The Trustee;
The Advocate;
The Representative

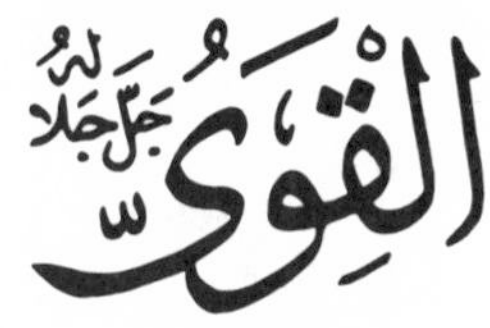

53. AL-QAWĪ
The Strong

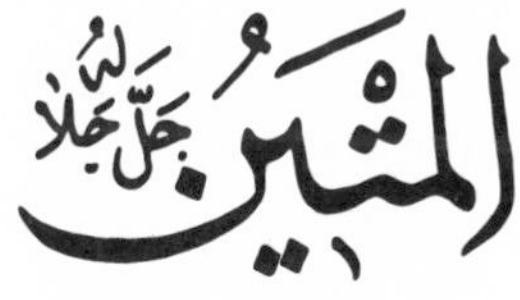

54. AL-MATĪN
The Firm;
The Steady

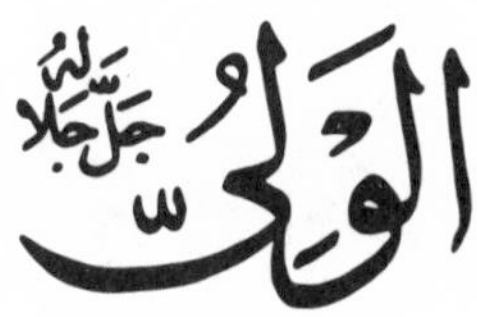

55. AL-WALĪ
The Protecting Friend;
The Patron

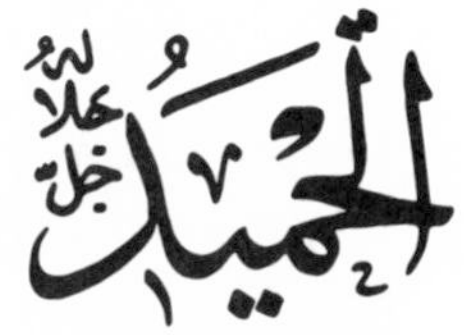

56. AL-ḤAMĪD
The Praiseworthy;
The Laudable

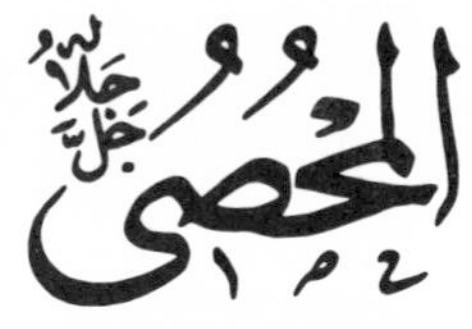

57. AL-MUḤSĪ
The Accountant;
The Counter

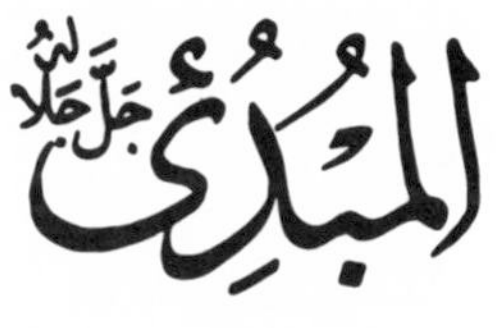

58. AL-MUBDĪ'
The Originator;
The Producer

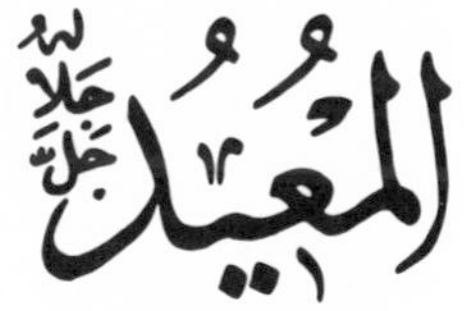

59. AL-MUᶜĪD
The Reproducer;
The Restorer

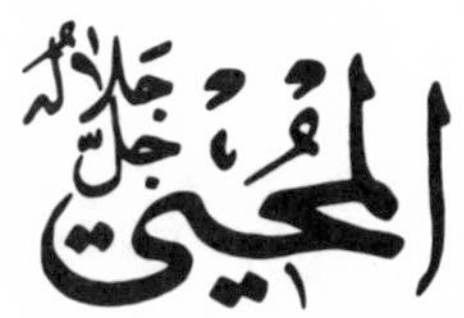

60. AL-MUḤYĪ
The Quickener

المميت جل جلاله

61. AL-MUMĪT
The Causer of Death;
The Destroyer

الحي جل جلاله

62. AL-ḤAYY
The Ever-Living;
The Alive

القيوم جل جلاله

63. AL-QAYYŪM
The Eternal;
The Self-Subsisting

الواجد جل جلاله

64. AL-WĀJID
The Illustrious;
The Noble

الماجد جل جلاله

65. AL-MĀJID
The Glorious

الواحد جل جلاله

66. AL-WĀḤID
The Unique

الأحد جل جلاله

67. AL-AḤAD
The One

الصمد جل جلاله

68. AṢ-ṢAMAD
The Eternal Support of Creation

القادر جل جلاله

69. AL-QĀDIR
The Able;
The Capable

المقتدر جل جلاله

70. AL-MUQTADIR
The Prevailing;
The Dominant;
The Powerful

المقدم جل جلاله

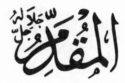

71. AL-MUQADDIM
The Promoter;
The Expediter;
The Bringer-Forward

المؤخر جل جلاله

72. AL-MU'AKHKHIR
The Deferrer;
The Retarder;
The Postponer

الأول جل جلاله

73. AL-AWWAL
The First

الآخر جل جلاله

74. AL-AKHIR
The Last

الظاهر جل جلاله

75. AẒ-ẒĀHIR
The Manifest;
The Outward

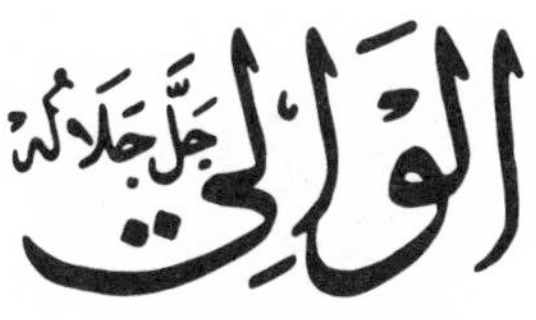

76. AL-BĀṬIN
The Hidden;
The Inward

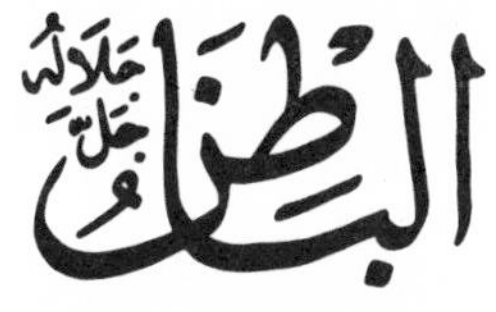

77. AL-WĀLĪ
The Governor

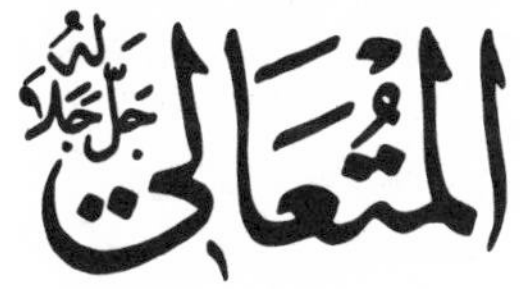

78. AL-MUTA^C^ĀLĪ
The High Exalted

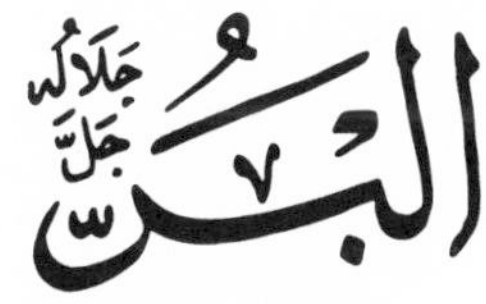

79. AL-BARR
The Righteous

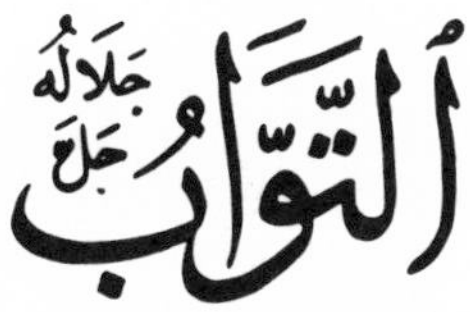

80. AT-TAWWĀB
The Accepter of Repentance;
The Relenting

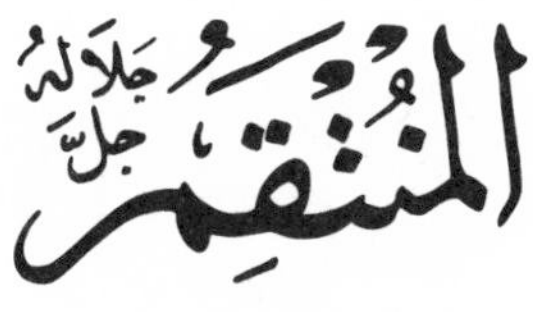

81. AL-MUNTAQIM
The Avenger

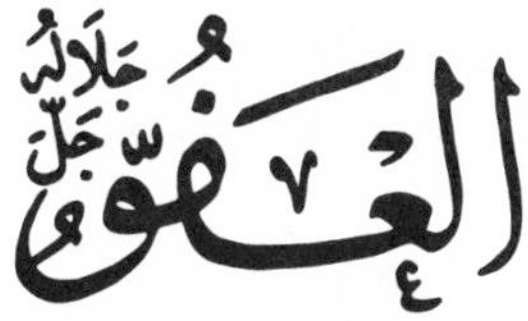

82. AL-^C^AFŪ
The Pardoner;
The Undulgent;
The Mild

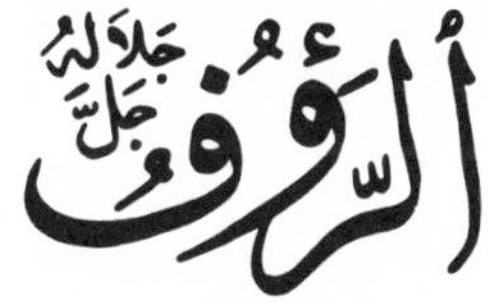

83. AR-RA'ŪF
The Compassionate;
The Full of Pity

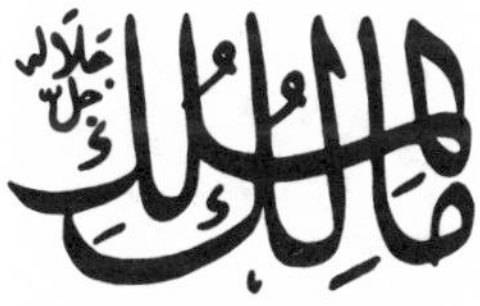

84. MĀLIK AL-MULK
The Owner of Sovereignty

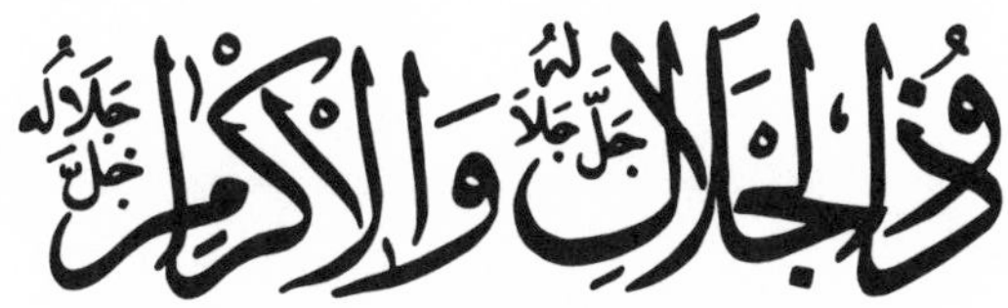

85. DHŪL-JALĀLI WAL-IKRĀM
The Lord of Majesty and Bounty

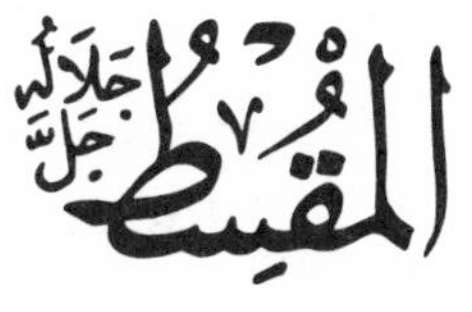

86. AL-MUQSIT
The Equitable

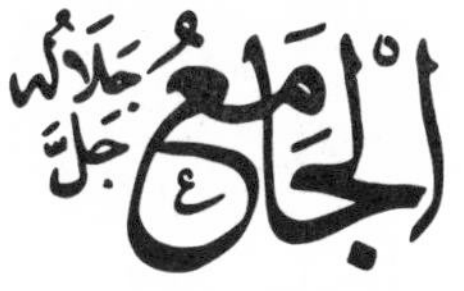

87. AL-JĀMI^C^
The Gatherer;
The Collector

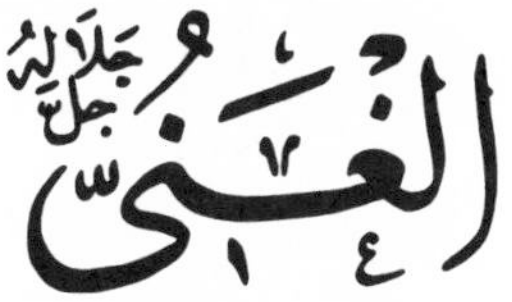

88. AL-GHANĪ
The Self-Sufficient;
The Rich;
The Independent

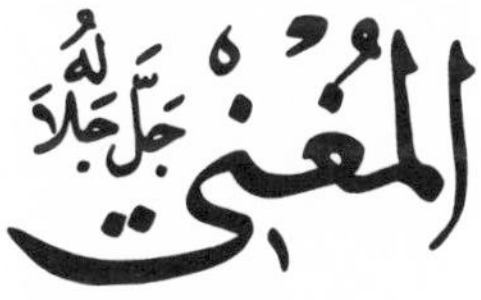

89. AL-MUGHNĪ
The Enricher

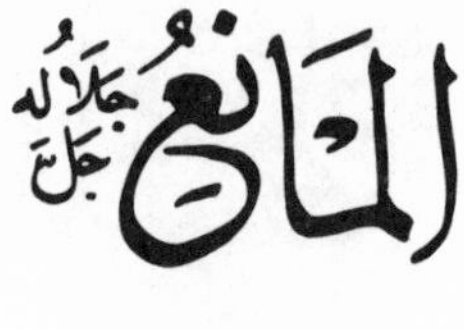

90. AL-MĀNI^c^
The Withholder;
The Preventer

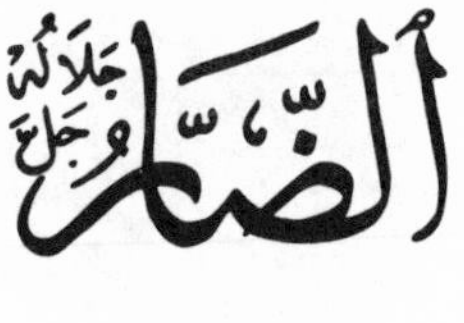

91. AḌ-ḌĀR
The Distresser

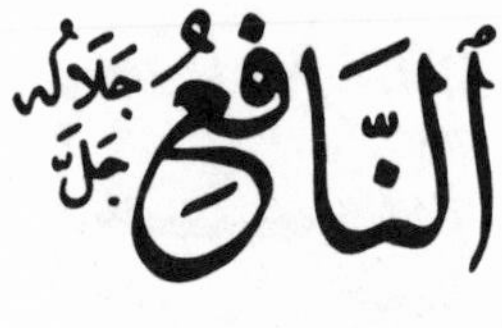

92. AN-NĀFI^c^
The Profiter;
The Propitious

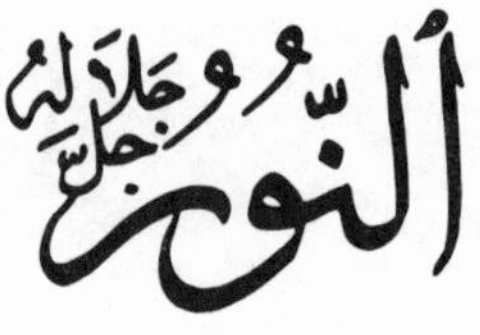

93. AN-NŪR
The Light

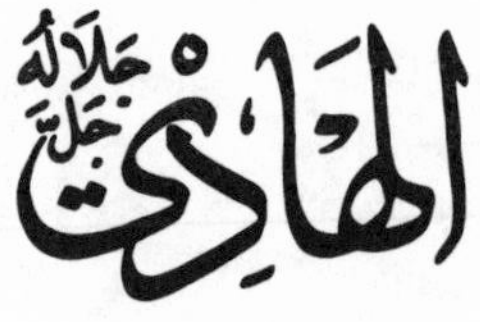

94. AL-HĀDĪ
The Guide

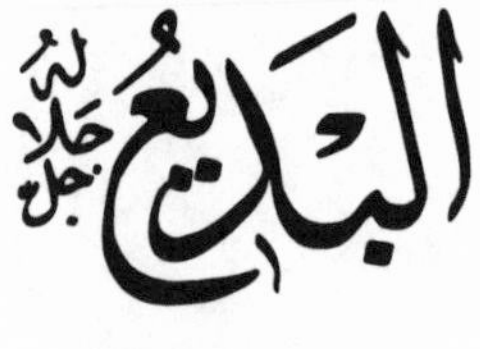

95. AL-BADĪ^c^
The Originator;
The Inventor;
The Incomparable

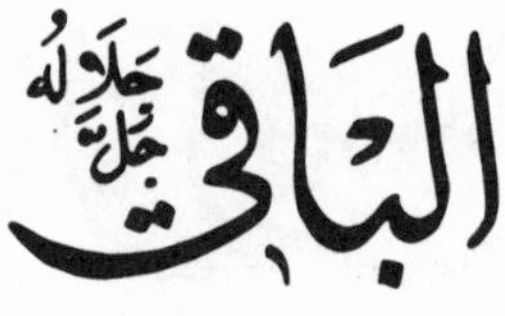

96. AL-BĀQĪ
The Everlasting;
The Enduring

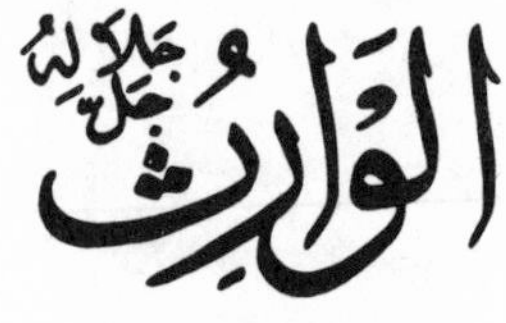

97. AL-WĀRITH
The Heir;
The Inheritor

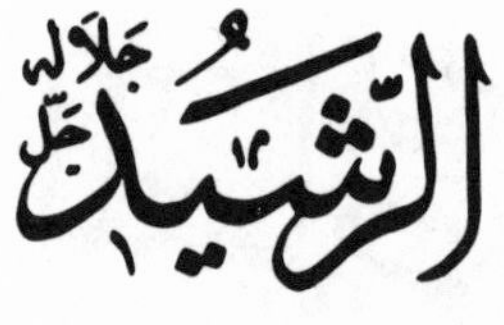

98. AR-RASHĪD
The Guide to the Right Path;
The Director

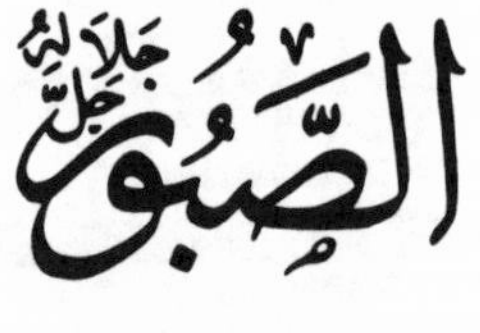

99. AṢ-ṢABŪR
The Patient

IV
Glossary

Abjad—Also called *jafr*; the science of numerical value configurations of the Arabic alphabet.

Akhlāt (sing. *khilṭ*)—Essences; humors; temperaments.

Allāh—The Arabic proper noun for the One True God (*al-ilah*: the Divinity).

Āmīn—"Be it so." Recited at the conclusion of prayers and supplications.

ᶜAql—Creative reasoning; reasoning power; the mind.

ᶜArsh—The Throne of Allah; the Ninth Heaven.

a.s.—Abbreviation of *ᶜalayhi as-salām*, "peace be upon him," the benediction invoked when the name of a prophet is mentioned.

ᶜAsr—The midafternoon obligatory prayer (*ṣalāt*).

Attar—An expressed true oil of a flower, wood, or bark, said to contain the essence of its soul.

Bismi Llāh ir-Raḥmān ir-Raḥīm—"In the Name of God, Most Gracious, Most Merciful"; the opening words of the Qur'an, frequently used as an invocation at the commencement of any word or action.

Chilla—A secluded room for spiritual practices; a forty-day retreat.

Dargah—A spiritual shrine or meeting place for living Sufi masters.

Dayo paree—Ghosts.

Ḍammah—A mark used in the Arabic language to denote the long vowel sound of *u*.

Dhikr (also spelled *zikr*, which signifies the Turkish and Persian pronunciation)—"Remembrance"; the Sufi ceremonies of liturgical recitations of sacred formulas and divine names.

Fajr—The predawn obligatory Islamic prayer; the time for this prayer.

Fanā'—Annihilation; effacement; passing away.

Fatḥah—A mark used in the Arabic language to denote the long vowel sound of *a*.

al-Fātiḥah (The Opening)—The first chapter of the Qur'an, said to concentrate within itself the whole Qur'an.

Fikr—The world of thought; deep meditation; remembrance of God by mental means.

Furjah—The human kingdom; the fourth interspace in the hierarchy of creation.

Garmi (Persian)—"Warm"; term used in reference to the metabolic values of foods.

al-Ghafūr (The Forgiver)—One of the divine attributes.

Ghayb—The Unseen as described in the Qur'an; includes the worlds of jinns, angels, disembodied souls, and other planes of existence.

Hadith (or *ḥadīth*)—A report embodying a *sunnah* of the Prophet (s.a.w.s.) or of the early Muslim community.

Ḥakīm—"Wise"; a physician who treats physical, mental, and spiritual illnesses.

Ḥaqīqah (or *ḥaqīqat*; from *ḥaqq*, "truth")—One of the four degrees of mystic experience in Sufism; the divine reality.

Himmah—Meditation; concentrated attention.

Ḥujrah—A shaykh's meditation cell.

Iḥsān—"Blessing"; the interior or internal conditions that result from performance of Islamic behaviors.

ᶜIlm—Knowledge.

Īmān—Faith in God.

Insān—The created world; life; human being.

ᶜIshā—The nighttime, or fifth, obligatory Islamic prayer of the day.

Islām—"Submission," "peace"; the way of life contained in the doctrines of the Qur'an and suggested in the statements and actions of the Prophet Muhammad (s.a.w.s.)

Idhn—The permission of God.

Jinn—A creation of Allah, made of smokeless fire; regulated by order of the Qur'an.

Kaᶜbah—The precincts of the Holy House, the first place of worship built by the prophet Abraham (a.s.) for worship of the one God; located at Mecca, Saudi Arabia.

Karāmah—A miraculous experience instigated by a Sufi shakykh. (See also *muᶜjizah*.)

Kaṣrah—A mark used in the Arabic language to denote the short vowel sound of *i*.

Khanaqah—A building used for spiritual retreat and training, usually occupied by three classes: people of seclusion, people of society, and travelers.

Lā ilāha illā Llāh, Muḥammadun rasūlu Llāh—The *kalimah* or Muslim profession of faith, translated: "There is no deity except Allah (God); Muhammad is the Messenger of God.

Mā shā' Allāh—"May it please Allah"; alternately,"As it pleases Allah."

Maᶜrifah (or *maᶜrifat*)—One of the conditions of Sufi experience, in which one is granted a glimpse of the divine reality; the knowledge that exists is that state.

Majdhūb—One experiencing the state of divine intoxication.

Mahal—House or level.

Maghrib—The after-sunset obligatory prayer of Islam.

Malā'ikah (sing. *malak*)—Angels.

Maqām—Stopping or resting place; station; stage.

Miswāk—A type of twig from the pelu tree recommended for brushing the teeth and cleansing the mouth. (Sometimes a licorice or olive tree twig is substituted.)

Mu^c^jizah—A divine miracle, which admits of no human activity or agency; an act beyond natural laws and reasoning power.

Murīd—A novice; a student of a shaykh.

Murshid—Guide; a Sufi shaykh; teacher.

Muslim—One who adopts and follows the way of life of Islam; a believer in God.

Nāfil—Superogatory or optional; distinct from obligatory (*fard*) worship.

Namāz (Persian, Urdu, Turkish)—*Ṣalāt*; prayer; worship.

Niyyah (or *niyyat*)—Intention; formal declaration to do something.

Nūr—The Light of Allah.

Nafs—The appetitive drives of the body, such as hunger, desire for wealth and fame, sexual urgings, etc.

Nafas—The breath of the spirit; pulse.

ᶜUd—An attar or essential oil made from the wood of the aloeswood tree.

Qalb—Heart; mind; soul; choicest part; genuine; pure.

Qiblah—The direction faced when offering Islamic prayers; the direction, from wherever one may be, facing the Kaᶜbah at Mecca.

Qiyām—One of the postures of *ṣalāt*, assumed by standing straight, with hands either held down at the sides or folded right hand over left and held just below the navel.

Qur'an—"Recitation"; the revealed scripture of the Islamic faith, conveyed by the angel Gabriel (a.s.) to the Prophet Muhammad (s.a.w.s.) over a period of twenty-three years.

Qurb—Nearness; proximity; approach; neighborhood.

r.a.—Abbreviation of *raḥmatu Llāh alayhi*, a phrase meaning "May the blessing of Allah be upon him," the benediction invoked when the name of any deceased Sufi is mentioned.

r.a.a.—Abbreviation of *raḍiy Allāhu ᶜanhu*, "May Allah be pleased with him," the benediction invoked when the name of a Companion of the Prophet is mentioned.

Raᶜkat (or *rakᶜah*)—One unit of the *ṣalāt*, Islamic prayer.

Ramaḍān—An Islamic month, signifying the days when the initial scriptures were sent down by God, including the Qur'an; the Islamic month of fasting.

Rasūl Allāh—The Messenger of God (s.a.w.s.); the Prophet Muhammad (s.a.w.s.).

Rūḥ—The soul; essence; breath of God; revelation.

Rukūᶜ—One of the postures of Islamic obligatory prayer, assumed by bending at the waist with hands placed upon knees.

Ṣalāt—The five-times-per-day obligatory Islamic prayer.

Sajdah—The posture of prostration in the Islamic prayer.

Samā'—Heaven.

*Samā*ᶜ—Ecstatic contemplation; audition.

Sardi (Persian)—"Cold"; term used in reference to the metabolic values of foods.

Shaykh—Sufi master; guide; teacher.

Shajarah—The listing of the names of shaykhs of a *silsilah*.

*Sharī*ᶜ*at* (or *sharī*ᶜ*ah*)—The divine laws and codes for human life, conveyed by all prophets, but corrected and completed and sealed in the first of the Last Message, the Holy Qur'an.

Silsilah—Line of transmission from master to master of the spiritual power and teaching of a *ṭarīqat*.

aṣ-Ṣiraṭ al-mustaqīm—The straight path; the path of right guidance ordained by the Holy Qur'an.

Sirr—Divine secrets; the greatest mystery; root; origin.

Ṣiyām—A fast, particularly the Islamic fast conducted during the month of Ramaḍān.

Subḥān Allāh—"All Praise belongs to Allah."

Sunnah—The behaviors (sometimes including the reports of others regarding Islamic life) performed by the Prophet Muhammad (s.a.w.s.).

Sūrat (or *sūrah*)—One chapter of the Qur'an. The Holy Qur'an is composed of 114 *sūrahs* of varying length.

Ṭarīqat (from *ṭariq*, "path")—The Sufi path; a stage of development in Sufism.

*Ta*ᶜ*wīdh*—A written or spoken religious amulet containing verses (and sometimes numbers) from the Holy Qur'an; frequently constructed by shaykhs for healing purposes.

Wahm—Imagination; the power of conceiving what is not present; the decision of Allah.

Walī (pl. *awliyā'*)—Friend of God; saint.

Waqf—A pause for breath marked in a written copy of the Qur'an.

Wiṣāl—Union; wedding; unity.

Yā Ḥayyu! Yā Qayyūm!—Literally, "O the Living! O the Ever-Lasting!" According to some Sufis, these two attributes together comprise the Greatest Name of Allah.

Yawm al-Qiyāmah—The Day of Judgment.

V
Bibliography

Abdullah, Mawlawi, and Maulawi Ala'addin (eds.). *Mizan-ul-tibb* (in Persian). Bombay: Haidari Press, n.d.

Al-Ghazzali. *The Mysteries of Fasting*. Lahore: Ashraf Press, 1968.

———. *The Mysteries of Purity*. Lahore: Ashraf Press, 1970.

Ali, A. Yusuf. *The Meaning of the Illustrious Qur'an*. Lahore: Ashraf Press, 1967.

Ali, Sufi Abu Anees Muhammad Barkat. *Makshoofat-e-manazal-e-Ehsan*, vols. I & II (trans. from Urdu into English by Muhammad Iqbal). Dar-ul-Ehsan, Faisalabad, Pakistan: Dar-ul-Ehsan Publications, 1978.

Balkhi, Sultan Ulema Bahauddin Walid. *Kitab-ulma'arif*. Manuscript, 13th century.

Balkhi, Mawlana Jelaluddin Rumi. *Masnavi*. Manuscript, 16th century.

Begg, Mirza Wahiduddin. The Big Five of India in Sufism. Ajmer, India: W. D. Begg, 1972.

———. *The Holy Biography of Hazrat Khwaja Muinuddin Chishti*. Tucson: The Chishti Order of America, 1977.

———. *The Holy Biography of Hazrat Khwaja Muinuddin Chishti* (Indian Edition). Ajmer, India: W. D. Begg, 1968.

Dehlvi, Hazrat Maulana Ahmad Saeed. *Prophetic Medical Sciences* (*The Savior*). Delhi: Arshad Saeed, 1977.

Eaton, Richard M. "The Shrine of Baba Farid in Pakpattan, Multan Suba'." Paper delivered at Association for Asian Studies Conference, Los Angeles, Calif., April 1, 1979.

El-Salakawy, Ahmad A. *Spotlights on Medical Terminology: The Human Body Systems* (in Arabic). 1972.

———. *Fundamentals of Medical Terminology* (in Arabic). Dar al-Maaref, Cairo, Egypt, 1968.

Elgood, Cyril (trans.). Tibb-ul-Nabbi or Medicine of the Prophet, being a Translation of Two Works of the Same Name—I. *The Tibb-ul-Nabbi of al-Suyuti*. II. *The Tibb-ul-Nabbi of Mahmud bin Mohamed al-Chaghhayni, Together with Introduction, Notes & Glossary*. Publication data not available.

Ewing, Katherine. "The Sufi as Saint, Curer and Exorcist in Modern Pakistan." Paper delivered at Association for Asian Studies Conference. Los Angeles, Calif., April 1, 1979.

Gohlman, William E. *The Life of Ibn Sina*. New York: State University of New York Press, 1974.

Gruner, O. Cameron, M.D. *A Treatise on the Canon of Medicine of Avicenna, Incorporating a Translation of the First Book*. New York: Augustus M. Kelly, 1970.

Hashmi, El Sheikh Syed Mubarik Ali Jilani. *An Introduction to Psychiatry*, Based on Teachings of the Holy Quran and Practice; Also Contains Results of Scientific Demonstration of Curing Incurable Mental Diseases in the Psychiatric Institute Taif, Saudi Arabia—1976–77. Lahore: Zavia Books, 1978. Revised 1979 and 1981.

Ibn Sina, *Qamus al-qanun fi'l-tibb*, New Delhi: Idarah ta'rikh al-tibb wa'l-tahqiq al-tibbi, 1967.

Kamal, Dr. Hassan. *Encyclopedia of Islamic Medicine*. Cairo: General Egyptian Book Organization, 1975.

Karim, Alhaj Maulana Fazlul. *Gazzqali's Ihya ulum-id-din, or The Revival of Religious Sciences, The Book of Constructive Virtues*, Part I. Dacca, Pakistan: F. K. Islam Mission Trust, 1971.

Khan, Dr. Muhammad Muhsin Khan (trans.). *Sahih al-bukhari*, vols. 1–12. Al-Medina al-Munauwara, Saudia Arabia: Islamic University, 1974. Revised 1976.

Khan, Sayed Mohammad Husain. *Qarabaadin-e kabir* (in Persian). Bombay: Munshi Nool, n.d.

Lawrence, Bruce B. "Healing Rituals among North Indian Chishti Saints of the Delhi Sultanate Period." Paper delivered at Conference of the Association for Asian Studies Conference. Los Angeles, Calif., April 1, 1979.

Levey, Martin, and al-Khaledy. *The Medical Formulary of al-Samarqandi and the Relation of Early Arabic Simples to Those Found in The Indigenous Medicine of the Near East and India*. Philadelphia: University of Pennsylvania Press, 1967.

Macey, Ann; Pam Hunte; and Hassian Kamiab. *Indigenous Health Practitioners in Afghanistan*. Kabul: Ministry of Public Health, 1975.

Nicholson, R. A. (trans.). *Kashf al-Mahjub of al-Hujwiri*. London: Luzac & Co., 1970.

Nizami, Ashraf F. *Namaz: The Yoga of Islam*. Baroda, India: Ashraf F. Nizami, 1976. Revised 1977.

Pelt, J. M., and J. C. Younos. "Plantes medicinales et drouges de l'Afghanistan." Extract from Bulletin de la Société de Pharmacie de Nancy, no. 66 (September 1965).

Quasem, Muhammad Abul. *The Jewels of the Qur'an, al-Ghazali's Theory*. Selangor, Malaysia: Dr. M. A. Quasem, 1977.

Rashid, Abdul; Mohammad Azam; Ahmad Jan; and Mohammad Ibrahim. *Rahat-ul-atfal* (in Persian). Kabul: Government Printing House, Reign of Habibullah.

Schimmel, Annemarie. *Mystical Dimensions of Islam*. Chapel Hill: University of North Carolina Press, 1976.

Shafii, Mohammad, M.D. "Adaptive and Therapeutic Aspects of Meditation." *International Journal of Psychoanalytic Psychotherapy* 2, no. 3 (1973).

———. "Light, Biological Rhythm and Integration of Personality in Sufi Meditation." Unpublished paper.

Siddiqi, ᶜAbdul Hamid (trans.). *Sahih Muslim*, vols. 1–4. Lahore: Ashraf Press, 1976, 1978.

Sprenger, Aloys, M.D. *Abdu-r-Razzaq's Dictionary of Technical Terms of the Sufis*. Lahore: Zulfiqar Ahmad, 1974.

Suhrawardi, Shaikh Shahaab-ud-Din ^{c}Umar b. Muhammad. *The ^{c}Awarif-ul-ma^{c}arif*. Lahore: Ashraf Press, 1973.

Tabibi, Dr. Abdul H. *Sirr-i tassawuf-i Afghanistan* (in Persian). Kabul: Ministry of Information and Culture, 1977.

Thomson, Robert, N.D. *Natural Medicine*. New York: McGraw-Hill Book Co., 1978.

———. *The Grosset Encyclopedia of Natural Medicine*. New York: Grosset & Dunlap, 1980.

———. *A Handbook of Common Herbal Remedies*. Orem, Utah: BiWorld Publishers, 1981.

———."Application of Tibb-ul-Nabbi to Modern Medical Practice." *Journal of the Islamic Medical Association* (Trenton, N.J.), vol. 11, nos. 1 & 2 (April 1980).

———. "Medicines for the Soul." Unpublished manuscript.

Valiuddin, Dr. Mir. *Contemplative Disciplines in Sufism*. London: East-West Publications (U.K.) Ltd., 1980.

———. *The Qur'anic Sufism*. Delhi: Motilal Banarsidass, 1959. Revised 1977.

Zamani, M. H. Saheb, Ph.D. (ed.). *Khat-i sewwom* (The Personality, Sayings, and Thoughts of Shams-e Tabrizi). Tehran: Atai Press, 1972.

Index

Administration, remedies, 67
Alcoholism, 28
Allergic reaction, 41
Alphabet, Arabic, 132
  and numerology, 132–135
  and regions of universe, 151–152
Amber, 115–116
Anemia, 68
Angels, 21
Anger, 28
Angina pectoris, 68–69
Animals, realm of, 20
Aniseed (*anīsūn*), 56
Appetite, corrupted, 30
Apple (*tuffāḥ*), 56
Application, of essential oils, 119–122
Arabic alphabet, 132–135
  and regions of universe, 151–152
Arrogance, 28, 29
Arthritis, 69
Asparagus (*hiyawn*), 56
Asthma, 70
Atrabilious essence, 45
Attars, 113
Auto-intoxication, 30
Azrael, Angel of Death, 21

Babbling, 31
Banana (*mawz*), 56
Barley, 56
Basil, sweet, 56
Bedwetting, 70–71
Bilious essence, 45
Blindness, 28
Blood essence, 45
Body
  and appetites (*nafs*), 12–13
  essences, 43–47
Boils, 82
Bread, 56
Breath (*nafas*), universe of, 123–129
Breathing, difficulty in, 32
Breath of life (*idhn*), 13–14
Bronchitis, in children, 71–72
Burns, 72
Butter, 56

Calendar, Islamic, 165
Cancer, 28
Carrots, 42–43, 57
Cauliflower, 57
Ceremony, *dhikr*, 143–146
Chamomile, 57
Chicken, 57
Children, bronchitis in, 71–72
Chlorides, 53
Chyme, 44
Cinnamon, 57
Citron, 57
Coconut, 57
Coffee bean, 57
Cold (ailment), 73
Cold, food, 41, 43–44, 48
Colic, 72–73
Common cold, 73
Concentration, lack of, 28
Constipation, 74
Coriander seed, 57
Cough, 74–75
Creation, hierarchy of, 17–23
Criminal behavior, 28
Crystalline heaven, 22
Cucumber, 58
Cumin, 58

Dates, dried, 58
Depression, 28
Devils (*shayatin*), 33
Dhikr, divine remembrance, 141–147
Diabetes, 75
Diarrhea, 29, 75–76, 88, 89
Digestion, 39–44
Divine attributes, 171
Divine remembrance (*dhikr*), 141–147
Divine secrets, station of (*maqām as-sirr*), 25, 30–32
Dosage, remedies, 66
Drug abuse, 28
Dysentery, 76

Earthly life, lack of interest in, 31
Ecstasy, 28
  excessive, 32
Eggplant, 58
Eggs, 58
Egotism, station of (*maqām an-nafs*), 25, 27–28
Eighth heaven, 22
Elemental spheres, 17–20
Eleventh heaven, 22
Empyrean, 22
Endive, 58
Enzymes, 44
Essences
  body, 43–50
  flowers, 111–122

Essential oils, 113
  application, 119–122
Eye problems, 28

Failure, fear of, 28
Fast days, 89
Fasting (*ṣiyām*), 85–90
Fatigue, 30
Fenugreek, 58
Fever, 29, 30, 32, 88, 89
Fig, 58
Fish, 59
Flowers, medicinal, 111–122
Flu, 41
Food
  eating, 43
  and health, 39–43
  metabolic values, 48
  preparation, 42–43
  of Prophet, 51–64
  selection, 41
Forgetfulness, 28
Formulary, 68–83
Frankincense, 116
Frivolity, 29

Gallbladder, 29
Garlic, 59
Ghee, 59
Ghosts (*dayo paree*), 33
Giddiness, 29
Ginger, 59
Gums, inflammation, 79

Hair loss, 80
Headache, 29, 76–77, 89
Healing
  crisis, 88–90
  flowers and oils for, 111–122
Health
  and food, 39–43
  defined, 11–16
Heart (*qalb*), 14
  attack, 28
  burning, 31
  pain, 31
  station of (*maqām al-qalb*), 25, 28–29
Heat, food, 43–44, 48
Heavens, 17
  and Earth, Keys of Treasures of, 155–158
  realm of, 20–22
Hemorrhoids, 77–78
Henna, 59
Herbal formulas
  administration, 67
  preparation, 65–67
  storage, 67

Hina, 118
Holistic health, 12
Honey, 59
Humans, realm of, 20
Hydrochloric acid, 44, 53
Hypocrisy, 28
Hypoglycemia, 28

Illness, as cleansing mechanism, 11–12
Inconsiderateness, 28
Indigestion, 78–79
Infallible remedy, 159–162
Inflammation of gums and toothache, 79
Intoxication, divine, 32
Irrationality, 31
Irritability, 29
Israfīl, Angel of Resurrection, 21
Itching, vaginal, 82–83

Jannat al-Fardaws, 118
Jasmine, 118
Jaundice, 28, 79–80
Jinns, 21, 32, 33
Joy, 28
Jupiter, realm of, 21

Key(s)
  to Paradise, 142
  of Treasures of Heavens and Earth,
    155–158
Kidneys, 29

Lentils, 60
Lettuce, 60
Light of Himmah, 21
Lunacy, 30

Maqalad as-Samawati wal Ard, 155–158
Marjoram, sweet, 60
Mars, realm of, 21
Meat, 60
Melon, 60
Menstruation, painful, 81
Mental world (*fikr*), 12–13
Merciful prescriptions, 131–140
Mercury, realm of, 21
Metabolic values, foods, 47–49
Metabolism, 46
Michael, archangel, 21
Migraine, 29
Milk, 61
Mint, 61
Miracles, origin of, 149–154
Moon, realm of, 20
Musk, 117
Myrrh, 116
Myrtle, 61

Narcissus, 61
Nausea, 29
Nearness to Allah, station of (*maqām al-qurb*), 32–34
Ninth heaven, 22
Nosebleed, 88
Numerology, and alphabet, 132–135

Obesity, 28, 80–81
Oils, of flowers, for healing, 112–122
Olive oil, 61
Olives, 61
Onions, 41, 42, 61–62

Painful menstruation, 81
Parsley, 62
Peach, 62
Perspiration, 88
Phlegm essence, 45–46
Pistachio, 62
Planets, realm of, 20–21
Pomegranate, 62
Postures, of Prophets, 91–109
Prayers, over rose petals, 114
Preparation, remedies, 65–67
Prescriptions, merciful, 131–140
Pride, 29
Proximity to Allah, station of, 25, 30–34
Pure spirit, station of, 25, 29–30

Quince, 62

Ramadan, 86
Reason (*ᶜaql*), 20
Reasoning power, of humans, 20
Reincarnation, 21
Remedies
  administration, 67
  infallible, 159–162
  preparation, 65–67
  storage, 67
Remembrance, divine (*dhikr*), 141–147
Rhubarb, 62
Rice, 62
Rose, soul of, 111–122

Saffron, 63
Ṣalāt, 91–109
Salt, 53, 63
Sandalwood, 117
Saturn, realm of, 21
Sayings, of Prophet, 54–55
Scalds, 72
Scalp problems, 29
Scent, and cooking, 42

Secrets, divine, station of, 30–32
Self-deception, 29
Self-illusion, 30
Senna, 63
Skin eruptions, 29, 82
Sleeplessness, 82
Soul (*ruh marks*), 13
  disembodied, 21
  essence, 25–27
  of rose, 111–122
  station of (*maqām ar-ruh*), 25–37
Spinach, 63
Spirit (*nafas*), 13, 26
Starless heaven, 22
Stations, of soul, 25–37
Storage, remedies, 67
Sublunary world, 17
Suffocating, sense of, 32
Sugar, 63
Sun, realm of, 21
Surat al-Fatihah, 159–162

Taᶜwīdh, 131–140
Tenth heaven, 22
Thyme, 63
Toothache, 79
Toxicity, 29
Treasures of Heavens and Earth, Keys of, 155–158
Tremors, 30

ᶜŪd, 118
Ulcers, skin, 82
Union with Allah, station of (*maqām al-wiṣāl*), 25, 34–36
Universe(s), 22
  of breath, 123–129
  regions, and Arabic alphabet, 151–153
Urination, 88

Vaginal itching, 82–83
Venereal disease, 28
Venus, realm of, 21
Vermicelli, 63
Vinegar, 64
Violet, 117
Vomiting, 88, 89

Walnut, 64
Water, 64
Wedding of God Almighty (*wiṣāl*), 23
Weights and measures, 66
Wheat, 64

Zodiacal heavens, realm of, 20–22

Other titles of interest...

Muhammad

His Life Based on the Earliest Sources

By Martin Lings

"This is simply the best biography of Muhammad in English. Lings has based it on eighth and ninth century accounts—some translated here for the first time—from individuals who lived through these events, who heard and observed Muhammad. Meticulously researched and perceptively written, it leaves it up to readers to decide for themselves who was this noble, enigmatic, devout, and very human prophet who had such an impact on past and present world history." ***Whole Earth Review***

ISBN 0-89281-170-6 • $16.95 pb

The Way of Sufi Chivalry

By Ibn al-Husayn al-Sulami
An Interpretation by Tosun Bayrak al-Jerrahi

A highly respected Sufi saint and scholar of the tenth century, Ibn al-Husayn al-Sulami compiled this book as a guide to enlightened behavior for the spiritual aspirant. He records the teachings of renowned spiritual masters, as well as quotations from the Koran and Hadith that reveal the true meaning of compassion, love, friendship, generosity, and hospitality.

ISBN 0-89281-317-2 • $10.95 pb

Journey to the Lord of Power

A Sufi Manual on Retreat

By Ibn 'Arabi
Introduction by Sheikh Muzaffer Ozak al-Jerrahi

This is the first English translation of a twelfth-century text dealing with spiritual ascent. 'Arabi, whose metaphysical teachings have had a profound influence on both the Muslim and Christian worlds, describes the evolutionary path of the journey toward God. It is chiefly concerned with spiritual retreat, an advanced and potentially dangerous Sufi practice that aims at the attainment of the Presence of God through absolute abandonment of the world.

ISBN 0-89281-018-1 • $10.95